DID YOU KNOW THAT . . .

- The ancient Romans drank the blood of a raven to rid themselves of gray hair?
- Natives of Greenland eat a certain fish to produce pregnancy . . . in both men and women?
- Some slaves in the American South insured a woman's love by scratching her with a dried bullfrog bone?
- Americans apply cucumber slices to the face to freshen the look of the skin?
- A European treatment for nosebleeds was to tie a string around the little finger?

FOLK MEDICINE
CURES AND CURIOSITIES . . .

for plenty of fascinating facts and remarkable revelations!

Also by Edward F. Dolan
Published by Ivy Books:

ANIMAL FOLKLORE: From Black Cats to White Horses
THE OLD FARMER'S ALMANAC BOOK OF WEATHER
  LORE

FOLK MEDICINE CURES AND CURIOSITIES

Edward F. Dolan

IVY BOOKS • NEW YORK

Ivy Books
Published by Ballantine Books
Copyright © 1993 by Edward F. Dolan

All rights reserved under International and Pan-American Copyright Conventions. Published in the United States by Ballantine Books, a division of Random House, Inc., New York, and simultaneously in Canada by Random House of Canada Limited, Toronto.

Quotations from A CORDIALL WATER
by M.F.K. Fisher Copyright © 1961, 1981
by M.F.K. Fisher. Reprinted by permission of North Point Press, a division of Farrar, Straus & Giroux, Inc.

ISBN 0-8041-0908-7

Printed in Canada

First Edition: September 1993

Contents

INTRODUCTION

Folk Medicine: Past and Present

ASIDE FROM the saving of their souls and the honoring of their gods or their God, the people of earlier times saw the keeping of their health as life's most vital task. They knew full well that survival hinged on the state of one's well-being. Illness and injury could, with frightening alacrity, take away a family's living, food, and shelter. The importance of good health to our forebears, from prehistory onward, is clearly reflected in a number of vintage sayings, among them:

He who has health has hope,
And he who has hope has all.

Arabian proverb

He that wants health wants all.

Health is better than wealth.

Irish proverb

We moderns differ in no way from our ancestors in our concern for our health. We are painfully aware, even in our age of miracle drugs and splendid surgeries, that the job of staying healthy is a difficult and often impossible one. But this difficulty is negligible compared to the problems faced by our forebears. In their time, living conditions for most were anything but conducive to good health. From prehistoric days, there has been a formal medicine (my term for what is today called professional medicine), some of it superb—witness the surgeries known to have been practiced at the dawn of time, and, later, the Hippocratic insistence on careful attention to personal hygiene—but, until very recent times, too much of it was of little or no help because it suffered from a lack of scientific understandings and equipment. Consequently, its attempts to explain the cause of illness and then to treat the sick were riddled with ideas and practices that were grounded in superstition, magic, and mistaken theories. Additionally, as is often regrettably the case even today, much of the formal medicine of old was beyond the reach of many ordinary families—especially the poor family unable to afford professional care and the backwoods family living too far from physicians.

Out of this situation—out of doctors working in a scientific darkness (or, at best, a half-light) and out of people tending to themselves, their loved ones, and their neighbors—came the body of lore that we today call folk medicine. Still cherished and employed by millions worldwide, in both advanced and primitive societies, this is a remarkable medicine, a vast collection of effective and useless curative practices, genuine and worthless medicines, legitimate and empty beliefs, and a deep-rooted faith in magic that it shared with formal medicine for centuries.

It is a lore that took shape in a number of ways. For one, it borrowed many of its medications from formal medicine. For example, plants and herbs that are still trusted worldwide in folk medicine (and, in a striking number of cases, formal medicine as well) were known to and employed by the doctors of antiquity. More than two thousand years before Christ, the Sumerians of the Tigris-Euphrates region were healing with a wide variety of plants, some of them of genuine value. Among their number was thyme, which modern science recognizes as an effective cough suppressant. According to the Ebers Papyrus (named for its nineteenth-century discoverer, German scholar Georg Ebers), the physicians of ancient Egypt treated their patients with at least seven hundred drugs derived from plants and other sources. On the list was aloe, the juice of which is noted for its ability to regenerate damaged tissue, and which finds employment today in the care of radiation burns.

It is safe to say that accident, which has played a role in so many historical developments, also has a place in the growth of folk medicine. Consider this possibility: in the American Midwest of the 1800s, mothers liked to feed their children stolen milk when the little ones fell ill with a cold. The treatment may well have dated back to some mother, here or in Europe, who, when her young son was sniffling and sneezing, happened to give him some milk that had been "borrowed" from the farm next door and was then happily startled to see him quickly recover. It didn't matter to her that the boy may have been about to recover anyway. She had stumbled upon what struck her as a marvelous cure. Because survival depended much upon the sharing of helpful knowledge among family and neighbors, she overcame her embarrassment and whispered of her discovery to her dearest friend. From there, her wondrous news spread to the outside world and became a staple of the lore.

Many of the discoveries, unearthed by accident or by trial and error, eventually showed themselves to be without value. A case in point: for centuries, people sent their ailing loved ones crawling through a double-rooted briar, or bramble, bush. The bush was thought to house great powers because of its dual root system and was believed to be able to cure rheumatism, whooping cough, skin problems, colds, and an assortment of other ills. A common practice was to pass a sick child over or through the bramble. The procedure proved a disappointment for many a parent: witness the woman in the mid-1800s who wrote that she had taken her little son three times through a bramble on nine consecutive days (the magic import of the numbers three and nine will be explained in chapter six), but that his cough "isn't no better." It can only be concluded that, when healing accompanied the bramble treatment, it was by coincidence. Or perhaps the bramble worked by auto-suggestion and helped simply by making the patients think that their condition was improved. Incidentally, it will do no good to tell this to someone who still believes in the efficacy of the bramble rite.

On the other hand, a great many folk cures did, in time, prove to be of value. For example, at some undated moment in the past, someone got the idea that asthma could be eased by swallowing a handful of spider webs rolled into a ball. The treatment was long (and still is) a feature of folk medicine and, in 1882, was found to have medicinal value. In that year, research discovered the substance *arachnidin* in the web. It showed itself to be a fine antipyretic.

As with ancient formal medicine, much of folk medicine was initially based on one of man's earliest concepts of the cause of illness, a concept that, on the basis of studies made of primitive people currently living as their ancestors did eons ago, is known to have evolved in prehistory. The concept holds that illness comes when something bad is put into the body or when something good is taken out of it. The causal agents are gods, devils, evil spirits, imps, demons, and any other such being that comes to mind. Let a man somehow anger a god, and he can count on the annoyed deity sending the creatures of illness into him. Let him walk where evil spirits or demons or whatever lurk (and they lurked everywhere in antiquity), and he risks having them invade his body to sicken him by staying for a while or by making off with his strength, energy, or, the choicest prize of all, his soul.

To many a modern eye, this age-old concept is superstitious nonsense. But consider two points. First, the notion that invading demons and the like carry our illnesses seems not so far-fetched when the word "germs" is substituted for "demons"; suggested is an intuitive understanding of what to us today is a basic truth. Second, there is the impressive fact that the concept took shape at the dawn of time, when the human mind was yet an infant; when lightning was not an electrical phenomenon but the bewildering immensity overhead signaling its wrath for some reason; when the wind and the night were not the results of a planet turning on its axis, but the one the sometimes gentle, sometimes grieving, sometimes enraged breath of the unknown, and the other a mysterious and somber visitor; when indeed, all the world was a place of mystery. Thus viewed, the concept emerges as an intellectual and imaginative triumph, a mighty effort by the untutored mind to fathom what was, at the time, unfathomable.

No matter what one may think of the concept, it gave to the world centuries of both folk and formal medical cures. One, as we'll see as early as chapter one, was to drive the unwelcome visitors back out of the body with foul-smelling and foul-tasting medicines intolerable to their supposed sensitivities—medicines that the patient was made to swallow or to endure having poured up his nose or into his ears. It was common practice in a number of early societies to mix into otherwise sensible medicines anything from sulfur to animal entrails and human hair and feces.

Vestiges of this age-old approach to treatment remain with us today, not only in folk medicine but also among people who would pout at the idea of being thought superstitious. How many of us still harbor the notion, learned in childhood, that the best medicine is also the worst tasting?

Likewise, and again in common with early formal medicine, much of the lore was and is based on magic. Virtually every ancient culture, from the most to the least sophisticated, attempted to cure its sick with practices and objects thought to have a magical or supernatural import—chants, prayers, songs, rituals, charms, amulets, and animals revered as sacred. Magic will crop up repeatedly in the coming chapters, but, for the moment, let one amulet suffice as an example of its work. The amulet, which was widely used as cure for inflammations and fevers, bore the following inscription based on a mystical word familiar to us all. The belief was that, as the word slowly faded away over a period of days, so would the affliction.

Abracadabra
Abracadabr
Abracadab
Abracada
Abracad
Abraca
Abrac
Abra
Abr
Ab
A

Personal observation of the characteristics or physical appearance of an animal or some natural object played a role in magical folk treatments. The fish, for instance, served as a fertility and sex symbol in cultures worldwide, in part because of its phallic shape and its ability to lay an extraordinary number of eggs. As a result, the Indians of the Caribbean advised a man to eat a diet of fish if he wished to have an extended life with his sexual powers intact.

Transference, long practiced in formal medicine, became a major strategy in folk cures and remains one to this day. Several kinds of transference were liberally used, as they still are. A major one sent a malady out of the patient and into another being or object; equally popular was the theory that a person could be helped to a cure or protected from a health problem by taking on a desired characteristic of another being. And so, on the one hand, Irish old-timers who suffer from rheumatism hold the hand of a corpse to their affected limbs and, as the casket is carried out, shout, "Take my pain with you!" On the other, there is the ancient Roman strategy for returning graying hair to its original dark shade: drink the blood of the raven, to absorb some of the bird's black color.

All the factors that have gone into the development of folk medicine make it not only one of the world's most fascinating bodies of lore but also one of the most illuminating. In it, we can see the best and the worst in our forebears—their hunger to comprehend and explain the mysterious and frightening in their universe; their determination to survive in its hostile environs, and the inventiveness, self-reliance, and courage they showed in doing so; their ability to make connections, as fanciful as those linkages may have been, between such apparently unrelated phenomena as the gray hair nature gave us and the black feathers it gave to the raven; their selfishness and wiliness in attempting to pass on something they didn't want to someone else; and their intelligence and imagination, those soaring faculties that enabled them to invent fine medications and procedures at one end of the medical scale, and the very oddest and most baseless of superstitious treatments at the other.

The purpose of this book is to report on the various aspects of that lore, explaining whenever possible the values of certain of its medications and practices; commenting whenever possible on the origins of its myriad beliefs; and trying always to show the wondrous intelligence and imagination that loomed behind the finest and most mistaken and ludicrous of its ideas and methods. It is a lore that provides us with an unusual look at the people of the near and faraway past and, since folk medicine is still practiced throughout the world and since we are not separate from our forebears, but simply the latest marchers in the long parade of humanity, a very close look at ourselves.

Two last points must be made before turning to the opening chapter. First, folk medicine can be divided into two branches. One concerns the medications and practices that have been used by generations as self-cures and health protections in the absence of formal medical care or the reluctance, for one reason or another, to employ it. The other concerns the folk doctors who have long been at work in many societies. Most of the book will be devoted to the self-care on which so many families have depended. The final chapter will turn to the folk doctors, the men and women who have come down through the ages bearing such names as witch doctor, shaman, *curandero*, and the title that is the best known of all, medicine man. Their names may have a strange ring to them and their practices may be echoes of a distant past, but make no mistake—in their own way, many were, and are, as professional and as knowledgeable as the modern physician with a degree from the finest university.

Finally, I am not a medical man, but simply someone who is interested in all aspects of folklore. And so, I am in no way recommending the use of any of the remedies, treatments, and theories to be mentioned in the coming pages. I am writing about them out of my own interest and for the interest you may have in what is a truly amazing lore.

Edward F. Dolan

CHAPTER ONE

Of Sniffles, Coughs, and Sore Throats

WE HUMANS have been fighting the common cold since the earliest of times, probably from the very day it caused its first victim to sneeze and ache all over. The battle has been a frustrating one. In all the centuries since that first sneeze and ache, we've been unable to find a cure for this mundane but thoroughly miserable complaint. We've learned how to hold certain flu strains at bay with immunizing agents. But not the common cold. What we've learned instead is to accept it with the resignation expressed in the vintage counsel:

Treat a cold and it will go away in fourteen days.
Leave it alone and it will depart in two weeks.

This resignation is such that it has been voiced at times with grim humor; witness this French medical advice that the late M. F. K. Fisher cites in her charming *A Cordiall Water: A Garland of Odd & Old Receipts to Assuage the Ills of Man & Beast*:

One tall silk hat, one four-poster bed, one bottle of brandy. To be taken as follows: put the tall silk hat on the right-hand post at the foot of the bed, lie down

11

and arrange yourself comfortably, drink the brandy, and when you see a tall silk hat on both the right and left bedposts, you are cured.

Just as resigned, but more succinctly put, is the advice of the esteemed Canadian physician Sir William Osler (1849–1919):

No food. Bed rest. A good book.

Mingled with the resignation is a dash of confusion. With Dr. Osler advising "no food," what are we to make of one of the most familiar of old adages?

Feed a cold and starve a fever.

For many, myself included, this is one of the most bewildering of sayings. It seems to be telling us to do one thing with a cold and another with a fever. But, all too often, the cold is accompanied by a fever. So what are we to do? Feast or fast?

Actually, what we're up against here is a message long accepted as having two different meanings—either the one mentioned above or the warning that one behavior can lead to another—namely, that feasting when down with a cold can invite a fever that will then have to be starved. Personally, I think the latter makes more sense. As stated in an old axiom, it cautions:

Don't feed a cold lest you should next be obliged to starve a fever.

But all this is much ado about nothing. Dr. Bruno Gebhard, in *American Folk Medicine: A Symposium*, flatly states that the whole feeding-a-cold idea is false. He says that the axiom first appeared around A.D. 50 in the works of the Roman medical writer Aulus Cornelius Celsus and, after being challenged in later centuries, was finally disproved during World War II when research showed that the intake of food does not raise the body's temperature.

Despite everything from resignation and confusion to downright frustration, we've never given up the fight against the common cold. Physicians, medicine men, medical charlatans, some of the most distinguished figures in history, families, and individuals—all have joined the battle through the ages. As a result, formal medicine has given us antibiotics, antihistamines, decongestants, and analgesics. And as a result, generations of families who have had to tend to themselves have filled the folk medicine cabinet with countless home remedies.

FOLK CARE FOR THE COLD

Every country and ethnic group in the world has devised its fair share of remedies for the cold and its accompanying discomforts—fevers, coughs, and sore throats. What has come down to us is a fascinating collection of practices and medications.

Some Practices

Many of the practices are steeped in superstition. In their book, *The Midwest Pioneer: His Ills, Cures, & Doctors*, Madge E. Pickard and R. Carlyle Buley point out that, had you been a child on the United States frontier in the 1800s, you would have been given a blue ribbon to wear and made to eat your meals off a blue dish and made to take your medicine from a blue bottle at the first sign of a cold. On the painful side of things, you might have been sent crawling through a double-rooted bramble, or briar, bush that faced eastward. And, at some point, your mother might have decided it was time to push a live fish down your throat and then pull it out and return it to the water.

It's difficult to pinpoint the origins of these practices, but it can be said that the trust in the blue ribbon as a health safeguard and curative can be traced back to the fifth century B.C., when Jewish parents attached fringes of blue to their children's clothing. Centuries later, in the 1600s, British architect Christopher Wren wrote of knowing a nobleman who always wore a blue garter as a protection against gout. As late as our own century, many English children wore necklaces of blue beads to ward off colds.

And what of the "blue dish and blue bottle" treatments? While they may be descended from the age-old trust in blue, they seem more strongly connected with a health fad of the mid-nineteenth century. At that time, blue glass windows were something new and were charming people everywhere. Seeing cash in the situation, medical charlatans announced that the blue rays of the sun could do wonders for one's health and then turned a nice profit by peddling a blue glass screen that, they claimed, would cure diverse ills for the patient who daily spent some time lying beneath it outdoors. It's reasonable to assume that families out on the frontier, wanting to get in on this marvelous new device but unable to afford it, decided that something already in the home—a blue dish or bottle—would serve quite as well for their various ailments, the cold among them. These cures were forgotten soon after blue glass became commonplace.

As for sending you crawling through a double-rooted bramble bush, your parents would here be adhering to a centuries-old superstition. The double-rooted bramble is one that has simply sent one of its branches back down into the earth, with the result that the branch has been shaped into an arch. Our forebears, with their penchant for seeing the supernatural in any natural oddity, regarded this as a magical occurrence that endowed the arch with great powers, among them the ability to cure. In the eleventh century, the newer of the two roots was cut up into nine pieces and boiled in a milky broth that was said to end dysentery. Later, children and adults were sent over or beneath the arch to cure rheumatism, whooping cough, skin problems, and other ailments.

And why were you made to crawl through an eastward-facing bramble arch? The reason for this can be seen in the old practice of passing an ill child at dawn through a bramble that faced the rising sun.

The faith in the half-swallowed fish probably dates back to the various ancient cultures that revered the creature as one possessing sacred qualities. To them, it symbolized fertility because of its phallic shape, its prodigious egg-laying talents, and the sexual implication they discerned in its ability to swim through—penetrate—water. Possessing sacred qualities, it was thought to be "divinely charged" and thus able to heal a variety of ills. The belief that whooping cough can be cured by swallowing a live fish still persists in certain regions of the United States.

This is far from being the only ancient practice that remains in vogue today in certain European and American regions. As cases in point, you can add to it these two New England remedies:

> If you have a sore throat, whether caused by a cold or not, take one of the stockings you've worn all that day and tie it about your neck.

> Wear a piece of silver on a string around your neck if you want to avoid colds and other contagious diseases.

The stocking counsel is a remnant of the ancient view that illness is brought by little demons who invade the body. In the antique mind, some of these creatures lurked everywhere—in the dark corners of a room, under beds, on rooftops, in water containers, in the very air that everyone breathed—and were ready to pounce on anyone at any moment. Others were sent by the gods to punish the individual for some transgression.

To recover, one had to drive the creatures back out of the body—and how better to put them to flight than to concoct some evil-tasting or foul-smelling medication that they would find intolerable? The doctors in antiquity dreamed up some beauties—foods, liquids, and salves laced with animal entrails, bones, or skin; human or animal dung; sulfur; and decaying plant roots. The whole concept lingers on among those Yankee old-timers who still turn to their stockings at the close of a long and sweaty day, certain that no self-respecting demon will consent to hang about for the night.

The ancients, though wide of the mark in blaming it all on demons, were on the right track in suspecting that illness can be caused by an outside agency— something that can "pounce" on us from out of the air, a friend's breath, or a sick person's belongings. When we talk of an epileptic seizure, we're speaking as the Romans did; their word for epilepsy meant *caught* or *seized*. And we talk as a number of ancient peoples did when we speak of "catching cold."

The advice to decorate the neck with a piece of silver on a string is a leftover from the age-old idea of transference—the notion that one could avoid or be rid of an illness by passing it on to something outside the body. The New England advice holds that when the silver turns black, it is showing that it has absorbed whatever it was that would have made you ill. What is more likely is that the chemicals in the body itself do the trick.

The Medications

In the main, the folk medications consist of drinks, inhalants, poultices, liquid massages, and salves. Most have been concocted from trees, foods, and plants. Among the trees have been the lemon and eucalyptus. Honey has always been a respected medicinal food, with such ancients as the Egyptians prescribing it for the relief of sore throats once they had noted the soothing effect its mucilage content has on irritated throat membranes. The list of plants is long and includes such herbs as boneset, catnip, ephedra, and horehound.

Many of these folk remedies have provided genuine comfort and, to one degree or another, have helped to heal. But others, in common with so many modern medicines, have been revealed to be anything from mildly to downright dangerous if used unwisely or by the wrong person. Camphor provides a convenient example:

For centuries (more than ten in China) a fragrant oil has been extracted from the bark, trunk, roots, and branches of the camphor tree—and more recently from the leaves too—and has been processed into crystals. Had you lived in the United States or Europe a century ago, you would have worn a bag of camphor crystals around your neck so that their fumes could do battle with a cold and a variety of other ills. Had you been suffering a cold, asthma, or emphysema, you would have heated the crystals in hot water and then breathed in their fumes.

All well and fine—unless you had miraculously lived on to our time, when pharmacological research has shown that prolonged inhalation of the fumes can poison the patient. The same holds true—and even more so—when camphor oil is taken internally, as it was for years in both folk and formal medicine to treat epilepsy and heart disease.

But there's no need to worry when you hear that camphor oil is used in present-day cough drops, soft drinks, and candies. The poison in the oil has been removed.

A Sampling of Drinks

Now, beginning with three of the many drinks that, either rightly or mistakenly, are trusted as fine general cold cures, let's look at some of the folk medications that have made their way down to us and are still cherished both here and in Europe.

Mormon Tea: Place 1 1/2 ounces of the dried branches of the ephedra plant in a pint of boiling water. Let the tea steep for five to twenty minutes.

Mormon tea can help because the ephedra plant contains the substance ephedrine, which research has established as an effective decongestant. Mormon tea, however, is made of the American species of the ephedra plant, which contains only trace amounts of ephedrine and isn't as potent as the centuries-old tea brewed from the Chinese ephedra, *ma-huang*. On the other hand, this might be a blessing if you're among those who can't handle the way ephedrine increases the heart rate and raises the blood pressure. Medically, ephedrine is presently used for assorted respiratory problems—among them asthma and emphysema—and certain types of epilepsy.

The tea is widely thought to have picked up its name from the fact that the early Mormon settlers wanted nothing to do with coffee and black tea and used the ephedra brew as a convenient and pleasant substitute. Depending on where you were raised, you might also know it as cowboy or squaw tea.

Catnip Tea: Pour boiling water over dried catnip leaves and flowering heads. Let the mixture steep for a bit before drinking.

Like Mormon tea, catnip tea may prove of some help. Exactly what good it does remains elusive, but it may be that the tea lends a hand by relaxing you and helping to bring on sleep. The catnip plant contains an oil with a chemical structure similar to the sedative substances—the *valepotriates*—found in the valerian plant. Valerian-based drugs are widely used as tranquilizers in European medicine.

As far back as the time of Christ, both folk and formal medicine were drafting catnip to take on just about any health disorder you'd care to mention, from the deadly to the most trivial. Early doctors in several cultures used it to battle such life threateners as leprosy and cancer. At the other end of the scale, its tea was used—as it still is by many a family—to relieve not only colds but also gas pains, flatulence, and infant colic. Its sedative properties early brought it into service to ward off insomnia and nightmares.

Hot Lemon Toddy: Before going to bed for the night, sip one or more glasses of hot water containing lemon juice. It's a good idea to take the drink while warmly cloaked in a blanket and with your feet in hot water.

From personal experience, I'm among those who are convinced that lemon juice in water as hot as you can tolerate does wonders for a cold. But I find that physicians are divided in their opinion as to the drink's actual value. Some say that its vitamin C content makes it a fine cold fighter and that its juice eases throat problems and catarrh. Others contend that studies do not prove the vitamin to be an especially efficient remedy but indicate only that people who take small amounts of it daily show some resistance to colds. Perhaps all that can be said is that the hot drink relaxes and, when followed by a night under the covers, often induces a comforting, fever-breaking perspiration.

The lemon drink is advised for both adults and children. Adults, however, may wish to try the hot toddy with a splash of alcohol. I don't drink (not out of any moral qualm but simply because I don't like the taste of alcohol), but I have some friends who swear there's not a cold remedy to compare with downing one or two fingers worth of whiskey in steaming water just before turning in for the night. Wine is credited with doing quite as well, with hot elderberry wine long being a favorite choice. The relaxing properties in alcohol, plus the perspiration that follows the toddy, may or may not actually reduce the time that the cold is due to linger. But my friends insist that, at the least, the nightly toddy can make that time seem not so long—and who am I to argue?

Mai Thomas, in her book *Grannie's Remedies*, writes that her Welsh grandmother heard of men who claimed to cure their colds by wearing boots into which they had poured a half-gill of whiskey. The remedy may seem odd—and blasphemous to seasoned imbibers—but it is one that has long been trusted not only in Wales but elsewhere in Europe.

Perhaps these strategies aren't as odd as they sound. We rub salves and the like into the chest and back—and so why not the feet? As do the chest and lungs, they provide an easy access to the body. If you'd like to put them to the test, you might try an experiment with a treatment that was once used on smallpox victims in both Europe and America. Tie a few cloves of garlic to the bottom of your feet. That notorious odor will soon arrive on your breath.

Stuffy Noses, Coughs, and Sore Throats

Now, what can be done to relieve the stuffy noses, congested lungs, coughs, and sore throats that accompany the cold? For an answer, try this unequivocal reply from Mrs. F. L. Gillette and Hugo Ziemann in their 1887 volume, *The White House Cook Book*:

> For cold in the head, there is nothing better than powdered borax, sniffed up the nose.

In case you're wondering what a cold remedy is doing in a cookbook, Mrs. Gillette and Mr. Ziemann did not limit themselves to writing recipes. They provided advice on everything from tending bed linen and preventing mold on jelly glasses to caring for the ill.

Their admiration for powdered borax may have been well-founded, but for those who find little appeal in the idea of sniffing it up the nose, let us turn to another old folk inhalant. To clear the head and nose:

> Place fresh or dried eucalyptus leaves in a quart of boiling water and let steep for about twenty minutes. Then inhale the fumes for several minutes. You may also drink the brew.

The eucalyptus tree is native to Australia. Long before it made its way to the outside world, the aborigines there depended on it to handle a wide variety of health problems—from injuries and abscesses to colds and asthma. That they knew what they were doing was shown when nineteenth-century research discovered that the oil in its mature leaves, bark, and roots is an active germicide with antiseptic and astringent properties.

As an inhalant or a medication taken internally, eucalyptus oil is widely employed to relieve not only the symptoms of colds and asthma but also croup, bronchitis, and other respiratory ailments. It goes into many of today's commercial products—rubbing compounds, liquids, and lozenges—that work to clear the nose and lungs and to relieve upper respiratory problems.

Worldwide, the folk remedies for easing coughs are legion. Their ingredients are varied, with possibly the most famous of the lot being the herb anise, which has been trusted throughout the western world ever since Hippocrates of Greece gave it his seal of approval as a cough suppressant some 2,400 years ago. Though the ingredients are varied, they were in the past known or thought to be expectorants, throat soothers, or a combination of the two.

Many of the cough recipes that have come down to us are on the thickish side. A number of American Indian tribes used maple syrup not only for coughs but other chest complaints as well. In the southern United States and the Ozarks, a syrup concocted of honey, wild cherries, and the flowers of the mullein plant has long been trusted for relieving coughs. (And, horror of horrors, one folk remedy advises the patient to smoke mullein leaves to cure chest colds, coughs, asthma, and other respiratory problems.) An old Pennsylvania recipe calls for a half-pint of white vinegar to be joined with two fresh eggs and a half-pound of rock candy and then mixed until it becomes a thick syrup. For many years, people with itchy throats on both sides of the

Atlantic turned to a syrup made of the juice of the elderberry.

Various cough remedies are brewed as teas. The ancient Greeks and Romans stirred the leaves of the coltsfoot plant into hot water to make a tea they considered so effective that each culture gave the plant a name that meant ''cough plant.'' Far across the world, the Gros Ventres Indians of Montana boiled the top leaves of the sage plant and drank the resulting brew for coughs, colds, and tuberculosis.

As for the sore throat, the ancient Egyptians thought honey an excellent remedy. Many of the French in Louisiana still put their faith in a tea made of melted tallow or elderberry leaves. A venerable Indian treatment calls for some rye flour to be boiled in a pint of milk for fifteen minutes, after which the mixture is spread on two lily onions to make a poultice that is then applied, lukewarm, about the throat.

How well do these and other assorted cough and sore-throat remedies work? To one degree or another, most are helpful (and those that are not often work nicely as placebos). Both coltsfoot and mullein are effective because of their mucilage content. But anise, though still as beloved as ever in folk medicine, has been found to be not much more than a mild expectorant and is blended into today's commercial cough drops and liquids principally for its pleasant taste. Its licorice flavor masks the bitter-tasting ingredients in the preparations.

A WORD ABOUT FLU

Many of our forebears were able to distinguish between the common cold and that other ailment that resembles it in so many ways, yet is far more uncomfortable and dangerous. As a result, the folk medicine cabinet also contains a number of flu remedies. For one, there's the United States variation of the Welshmen's tactic of pouring whiskey into their boots to be rid of a cold. Here, flu was long fought by placing sulfur in the victim's shoes (perhaps on the grounds that the Welshmen were wasting perfectly good whiskey).

Eliot Wigginton, in *The Foxfire Book*, mentions a venerable and trusted prescription from the mountains of the United States southland. It calls for you to gather the leaves of the boneset plant and place them in a sack. Let the sack stay out in the sun for a time so the leaves can dry. There should be ample air circulation to keep them for turning moldy. Once they are dry, you're to boil the leaves with water, strain them off, and drink the brew.

The brew sounds pretty potent, but so far as modern research is concerned, there is a problem with boneset. There is no proof that the plant does a bit of good.

Boneset is native to America, and generations of early Indians, were they still alive, would likely insist that science has simply failed to unearth the proof of its efficacy as yet. Long before our first settlers learned of its wonders and sent the word, and some plants, back to Europe, boneset served as a trusted native cure for a string of complaints that ranged from constipation to typhoid fever and malaria, with snakebite thrown in for good measure.

And it would certainly do no good to tell the Americans and Europeans of the 1700s and 1800s that bone-set is without value. It was their premier remedy for colds, coughs, and flu. In fact, the plant came by its name because it was thought to be able to cure break-bone flu, a particularly vicious nineteenth-century malady that caused body aches severe enough to make its victims predict that their bones were going to "break any minute now."

PROTECTING AGAINST COLDS

Now, what can be done to avoid a cold in the first place? According to folk medicine, a host of defenses are at your disposal. For one, you can choose a once-popular European and American defense and go about your daily business with the pelt of a cat pressed against your chest. Until our own century, the pelt was thought to be a safeguard against the colds and chills brought on by damp and icy air. The idea was not, however, to provide an extra layer of protective covering. Rather, the practice stemmed from a superstition of the Middle Ages—that cats are immune to diseases of every ilk. In its turn, that superstition was likely an outgrowth of the ancient fancy that the cat, because of its agility and its talent for landing on its feet at the end of a fall, is blessed with nine lives. This notion is no longer taken seriously, but it does remain a part of our everyday language.

Also steeped in superstition is another avoidance tactic you might try, one that is still employed in the Ozarks and elsewhere. Simply tie a red onion to your bed. Or, as is still done in New England, you can carry an onion in your pocket. If you do, Yankee old-timers will tell you that you're due for an extra bonus. You won't get fits (epilepsy).

Both are echoes of that old belief about disease being the work of invading demons. Neither, however, drives the trespassers out of the body, but each holds them at bay and keeps them from entering it the first place with a pungent food (some choose garlic rather than the onion). Actually, many people looked on garlic and the onion as being able to do double duty. When worn on the person, either was thought to be able to stop the invasion of an illness and, at the same time, to soak up whatever there was of it that had already entered the body.

Had you lived in any of a number of societies, both ancient and recent, you would have kept illness and sick people at arm's length by wearing amulets containing not only strong-smelling plants but also any disgusting object you could think of. To prove the point, we need only remember one of the most infamous amulets of all time—the asafetida bag. Asafetida itself, with an odor that is anything but inviting, is a resin extracted from certain varieties of the fennel plant. It was carried for centuries in various parts of the world and was garnished with any substance that the people of a given time or place thought would increase its powers—ashes, dirt, rotting meat, bones, decayed plant stems and leaves. When worn about the neck, it was supposed to ward off not only all kinds of disease, but witches and evil spirits to boot. As late as our own century, countless Europeans and Americans had their childhood ruined by having to wear the bag as a health safeguard.

The asafetida bag is still carried in the pocket by

some Europeans as a protection against smallpox. It also continues to be used as a folk remedy for freeing infants of colic and keeping them in good health (you may take your choice as to whether it actually works on the little ones or simply proves that they were born blessed with steel constitutions).

Finally, to protect you and yours from colds, you can take to heart a pair of axioms on the dangers of icy, drafty, and damp air. Coming as they do from two widely separated nations, they leave no doubt as to how the common cold—not to mention other infectious ailments—has troubled people everywhere, no matter their time, no matter their place:

Back to the draft is face to the grave.

China

If cold wind reach througyh [sic] a hole,
Say your prayers and mind your soul.

England

COLLECTIBLES

On Doctors

Both folk and formal medicine abound with views and comments on the myriad facets of health and disease. There are so many, and they are so varied, that it is impossible to place them all within the topics that make up the chapters of this book. So that you can enjoy them and be intrigued by what they have to say, here is the first of seven collections of comments, beliefs, proverbs, rhymes, and the like that resist the idea of being contained within the chapters.

The collections will be placed between the chapters. With one exception—a set of contrastingly grim and pleasant conjectures on death—each will focus on some aspect of health and its upkeep. There will be brief explanations of those entries whose meanings are not immediately clear.

We begin with the world's doctors. The comments below leave no doubt that the physician has long been both the most maligned and admired of individuals.

If you have a physician for your friend,
Tip your hat and send him your enemy.

When one's all right, he's prone to spite
The doctor's peaceful mission.
But when he's sick,

It's loud and quick
He calls for the physician.

Doctors
Eugene Field

The doctor is often more to be feared than the disease.

It's no trifle at her time of life
To part with a doctor who knows her constitution.

Janet's Repentance
George Eliot (1819–1880)

If the doctor cures, the sun sees it,
But if he kills, the earth hides it.

A priest sees people at their best,
A lawyer at their worst,
And a doctor as they really are.

The physician's hope, every misfortune.

Ireland

No physician, in so far as he is a physician, considers his own good in what he prescribes, but the good of his patient; for the true physician is also a ruler, having the human body as a subject, and is not a mere money-maker.

The Republic, Book I
Plato (c. 427–347 B.C.)

* * *

One doctor makes work for another.

Young physicians fatten the churchyard

The comment here is that inexperienced doctors may be prone to making fatal mistakes.

And now some truths:

The best doctors in the world are Doctor Diet, Doctor Quiet, and Doctor Merryman.

Dialogue II
Jonathan Swift (1667–1745)

By medicine life may be prolonged, yet death will seize the doctor too.

Cymbeline, Act V
William Shakespeare (1564–1616)

The doctor is an angel when employed,
But a devil when one must pay him.

And the greatest truth of all:

It is no time to go to the doctor when the patient is dead.

Ireland

CHAPTER TWO

Beauty for the Eye
of the Beholder

Colds arrive periodically —far too often in every-one's opinion, yet still only on occasion. But we live daily with the world watching us and accepting or re-jecting us, much on the basis of what it sees. Knowing this, we, in common with all those who have preceded us, cannot help but be concerned with our physical ap-pearance. As a result, folk medicine boasts a treasure trove of practices and concoctions meant to keep us looking more attractive than nature intended and younger than we actually are. That it has produced so many is not surprising. Until the use of manufactured skin-care products became widespread among the av-erage family in recent times, most beauty aids were dreamed up in the home and passed from generation to generation.

Beginning with what has long been called "woman's crowning glory," let's see what has been done through the ages to help us please the eyes of our beholders.

HAIR

It's unfair to think only of women when describing hair as a "crowning glory." Quite as much as females, the males of the species have been taken for centuries with the idea of sporting a handsome thatch atop the head. For proof, we can begin with the extravagant male coiffures on view today. A drop back in time brings us, in turn, to the neck-length styles worn by the poet Shelley in the nineteenth century and Benjamin Franklin in the eighteenth; the flowing locks of the English Cavaliers in the 1600s; and the medical defense brought to bear against graying hair in ancient Rome. When the Roman doctor prescribed downing cups filled with raven's blood to retain or recapture the hair's original color, he was heeded by as many men as women. The treatment, of course, is a prime example of the theory of transference at work in medicine. Drinking of the raven's blood, as remarked in the introduction, was thought to impart the bird's black color to the patient's graying hair.

While we males prefer our hair in its original shade, we are far more preoccupied with keeping the stuff should it—as it has the deplorable habit of doing— decide to leave. Until the recent coming of hair transplants, formal medicine pretty well threw up its hands in the face of the inevitable. But not folk medicine. Over the centuries, it has dreamed up numerous remedies to stop or reverse the onslaught of baldness. Many remain in use today, ranging from the benign to at least two that require superhuman determination (or sheer desperation) and a cast-iron stomach on the part of the patient.

The former include a simple method for correcting matters when the hair is beginning to depart: we need do no more than wash our heads regularly in water laced with salt. Another—this one from ancient Greece— advises us to massage a paste made of the leaves of the aloe plant into the scalp. Still another is meant for those who, unable to stop the departure, now yearn for a new growth of hair: wash the head with water containing the leaves and flowering parts of the sage plant. This treatment was advised in Europe and came to America with the early settlers. Long before the newcomers arrived, however, the Montana Indians were using a similar restorer—water infused with blue sage or sagebrush. They said the mixture also worked well as a general tonic.

Now for the two requiring a strong stomach: the first is still trusted in the Ozarks and parts of the southern United States. We're to massage our balding heads with manure—*fresh* manure, God help us. The second involves the mole, a little animal that has played a role in folk medicine since Roman times and was once widely thought capable of curing just about anything. It recommends boiling the mole and then rubbing its flesh into the scalp. A variation advises massaging the scalp with the animal's blood. Wayland D. Hand, writing in *American Folk Medicine: A Symposium*, reports that the first of the two mole treatments was being used in Germany's Swabia region early in our century, while the second is employed in the mountains of North Carolina.

Should the manure (fresh, remember) and mole remedies require too strong a stomach, we can turn to a treatment that contains only a few unattractive ingredients and was recommended in 1887 by Mrs. F. L. Gillette and Hugo Ziemann in their eclectic *The White House Cook Book*:

HAIR INVIGORATOR

Bay rum, two pints; alcohol, one pint; castor oil, one

ounce; carb. ammonia, half an ounce; tincture of cantharides, one ounce. Mix them well. This compound will promote the growth of hair and keep it from falling out.

Tincture of cantharides is a solution containing the notorious Spanish fly in dried form. Spanish fly, which was once thought—and still is by many people—to be a powerful aphrodisiac, is made of the beetles of the *Cantharis vesicatoria* species. Today, it is known to be downright dangerous when taken internally. It irritates the genito-urinary tract, causes intense pain, makes urination difficult, and often produces blood in the urine. Ingestion of as little as 1.5 grams can kill—and has. Applied externally, it can blister the skin.

If the Gillette-Ziemann formula isn't to your liking, there's another old-timer waiting for a try: massage garlic into the scalp. Or how about concocting a plaster of boiled quince mixed with wax and spreading it over the bald spot? What you're attempting here is some transference, hoping that the fuzzy-skinned quince will produce something similar atop your head. Should all else fail, you can always fall back on the old European superstition that a thick mane will result if you allow a pregnant woman to give you a haircut.

But enough of baldness. Here are some folk treatments that both men and women can use in the hopes of improving the condition and looks of the hair. To be rid of dandruff, you can try the venerable European and southern United States system of washing the hair in warm borax water. For a luxury of curls, New England old-timers will likely recommend that you eat bread pudding and milk or, if that dish isn't to your liking, bread crusts. I suspect that the bread-pudding tactic may have gotten its start among mothers who were trying to tempt their youngsters, especially their daughters, into trying an entree not noted for its splendid look and taste. Cut from the same cloth was the parental encouragement of my own boyhood: ''Eat your spinach so you'll be strong like Popeye.''

For centuries, herbal rinses to give the hair greater luster have been used by both sexes. The herbs most favored for the rinses are chamomile (often spelled *camomile*), sage, and rosemary. Chamomile is recommended for bringing out the tones in lighter-colored or blond hair. Sage and rosemary, which can be used either singly or together, are best for darker shades. The rinses are made by simply mixing the leaves and flowering parts of the desired herb in water and then pouring the blend onto your head after shampooing. The rinses can also be added to your shampoo.

FOR A CLEAR COMPLEXION

May 28: After dinner, my wife away down with Jane and W. Hewer to Woolwich in order to a little ayre and lie there tonight, and so to gather May dew tomorrow morning, which Mrs. Turner has taught her as the only thing in the world to wash her face with, and I am contented with it.

Diary
Samuel Pepys (1633–1703)

Any woman who desires a clear complexion might wish to start with a dainty custom that has come down to us from the Scotland and England of at least three centuries ago. The maiden of that time was promised glowing skin and great beauty for the entire year—or, according to the beliefs in some districts, for all time to come—if she would go out early on May Day and rinse her face with dew water. In Scotland's Edinburgh, it was long the custom for young women (and men) to walk up the hill called Arthur's Seat, and there to "meet the dew" just before sunrise on May Day and guarantee themselves twelve months of both fine looks and good fortune. Lasting beauty in some areas could be had if the dew water was collected on the first Sunday in May. In fact, as Mrs. Pepys was out to do, one could benefit from gathering the water at any time of the month. It was reputed not only to beautify but also to erase blotches, smoothe out wrinkles, and hold at bay the first traces of advancing age.

Though we know today that dew is the result of condensation on a cold and clear night and that its disappearance is caused by evaporation, dew has always played a major role in folk beliefs. To people everywhere, it was a magical substance because it seemed to fall mysteriously from heaven in the dark and then vanish when touched by the sunlight. As such, it was widely employed in the formal medicine of the 1600s as a skin lotion. It was also prescribed for sore eyes and was thought to be able, if used in specific ways, to cure several other ills—for example, vertigo if sniffed up the nostrils, and failing sight if dabbed on the eyes after being collected from the leaves of the fennel plant.

Were you a young lady who missed the chance of collecting dew on May Day morning, you could avail yourself of liquids and pastes fashioned from any of various fruits, herbs, flowers, and vegetables. In areas of the southern United States, you could make a paste of bananas for gently massaging into the skin. In both Europe and America, you could allow the steam from boiling water, spiced with lavender flowers, dried sage leaves, chamomile flowers, or fresh or dried parsley, to flow over your face for a few minutes. Or, for what was long reputed to be one of the best liquid massages, you could place apple blossoms in a half-pint of water that was then allowed to boil down to a teaspoonful, after which it was to be poured into a half-pint of sherry wine.

Another liquid massage could be made by pouring boiling milk over violets. This was much trusted for whitening and softening the skin, and added an extra benefit as well. It helped to get rid of wrinkles.

The cucumber was—and still is—especially admired as a beauty aid both here and in Europe. To freshen the look of the skin, you needed to do no more than gently rub the face with cucumber slices. The massage could also be done with slices that had been soaked in rum.

How women first came upon the cosmetic value of the cucumber is unknown. What has been established is that, when eaten, the cucumber does have a happy effect on the skin because it cools the body and purifies the bowels and blood. It seems obvious that the skin will react positively when the vegetable is applied directly to it.

Now, in what certainly is a blatant contradiction of terms, we come to an unappealing substance that has long been highly recommended in many areas for producing appealing skin—human urine. I cannot resist turning this matter over to M. F. K. Fisher and letting her speak of it as she does in *A Cordiall Water: A*

Garland of Odd & Old Receipts to Assuage the Ills of Man & Beast. She writes that she first heard of the therapeutic values of urine when "my mother whispered to me that mixed with an equal part of water it would make smilax ferns grow long and beautiful. . . . She shuddered a little when she confided this to me. . . ."

And so, "Surely it was not from her, then, that I heard, also in whispers, that southern girls had the whitest skins in America because they patted themselves each night with their own warm urine, perfumed with lavender?"

The author then provides us with a bridge to our next topic by writing that urine will also get rid of freckles— at least according to a farm woman she once knew in Provence, France. "She suffered mightily from them when she was a teasable child, until her grandmother, who was mountainborn, gave her this recipe:

Take a wineglass of urine and mix it with a table-spoon of good vinegar. Add a pinch of salt. Let it sit for 24 hours. Then pat it on the freckled skin and leave it for one half-hour, and rinse off with plain cold water."

If, as is strongly suspected, freckles are caused by exposure to light, they have been pestering both young and old for as long as there have been people on the planet. In the past, they were a particular embarrassment for the young farm woman who had to spend much of her life outdoors. Consequently, folk medicine soon came forward with a variety of cures. Still in use today are such remedies as wearing nutmeg around the neck, dabbing the little spots with sap from a grapevine, and massaging them with a mixture of buttermilk and lemon juice.

One very popular European and American measure is assuredly an outgrowth of the Scottish-English method for insuring a fine complexion. This time, to be rid of your freckles, you're to rinse your face with that morning dew that is collected on May Day. A variation is seen in parts of the American South: you'll do nicely by washing your face with the water in a maple stump on that day.

Another variation advises you to gather morning dew (no special day is mentioned) and massage it vigorously into your freckles while reciting:

Dew, dew, do, do
Take my freckles
Away with you.
Dew, dew,
Thank you.

SORES AND ITCHES

Unless nature deems otherwise, a clear skin can be hard to come by, and, unless the fates deem otherwise, it can be impossible to keep unsullied at all times. There's not a one of us who, at one time or another, hasn't suffered insect bites, sores, boils, itches (from having eaten one too many chocolate candies or from stumbling into a patch of poison ivy), cuts, and scratches. Folk medicine has its cures for them all. The cures, as usual, range from the magical to the quite practical.

Consider first what would have been in store for you had you been a child of a century or more ago out on the midwestern plains, and had you fallen prey to the contagious erysipelas with its swellings and eruptions. In *The Midwest Pioneer: His Ills, Cures, & Doctors*, Madge E. Pickard and R. Carlyle Buley tell us that epidemics of erysipelas were common at the time and that the cures were several. For one, your parents might fetch home the mother of twins to help. She would strike a flint and steel over your head, with the hope that the sparks would somehow drive the disease out of you. Or your mother might place nine catkins from a birch branch on the swollen and inflamed areas of your skin. For the cure to work, she had to collect the catkins on a Friday morning—and she had to do so without speaking to anyone.

On the practical side of things, no matter where you lived, you would have treated sores, itches, and wounds of one degree or another with any of a number of plants. Among those widely admired for their healing abilities were the herbs comfrey, fennel, lavender, and wintergreen. Some examples:

In Europe, especially in France and Spain, bruises and insect bites were—and still are—treated by covering the affected area with a poultice containing the oil extracted from the flowers of the lavender plant. The treatment helps because of the antiseptic properties contained in the oil.

Folk treatments for sores and wounds in both Europe and the United States have long called for the use of potions or poultices concocted from the leaves, stems, and flowering parts of the comfrey plant. Ever since Greek and Roman times, this plant has been highly prized for its ability to heal the skin by quickly closing it over; in fact, its botanical name, *Symphytum*, means "grown together." In antiquity, comfrey was thought to be able to hasten the mending of broken bones, and its name is thought to have come from the Latin *conferve*, meaning "knitting together." There is no doubt that comfrey does help to heal blemished and injured skin. What makes it work is its allantoin content. Allantoin is a crystalline substance that affects the multiplication of cells and tissue growth.

Ever since the nineteenth century, a folk treatment here and abroad for someone who has blundered into a patch of poison ivy or poison oak has been to place the leaves, stems, and flowers of the grindelia plant in boiling water, allow the mixture to cool, and then apply it to the itching skin by means of a cloth compress. Thanks to a soothing resin in the plant, the treatment is said to work pretty well.

Another time-honored remedy for the agony of poison oak or ivy—and one that is also good for treating burns—is to coat the skin with juice squeezed from the aloe plant. Aloe has been admired as a healer since antiquity, with the Roman naturalist Pliny the Elder (A.D. 23–79) writing that its juice could be used not only for skin irritations but also for burns and wounds. His claims are justified in the recognition that modern science has given to aloe's ability to regenerate damaged tissues swiftly. Its juice is now used to treat radiation burns.

Our talk of skin problems brings us now to one of the most common and troublesome of the lot, one that has taken a backseat to no other so far as the number of folk treatments that have been devised for its riddance—the plain, everyday wart.

THE WART

The ugliness of this commonplace disfigurement has been annoying people everywhere since antiquity. At that time, it was thought to be caused by picking up and handling a toad. This belief, which has persisted through the centuries and remains intact today in many localities, was based on two characteristics seen in the little animal. First, there is the coincidental resemblance of the wart to the toad's rough, somewhat horny skin. Second, there is the fact that, when grabbed in the mouth of another animal, like a dog or a fox, the toad protects itself by exuding a fluid that irritates the captor's tissues and causes it to release its captive. From the earliest of times, one of the first lessons a child learned was to have no traffic with toads or (a case of guilt by association) their near relatives, frogs.

Most of the wart cures that have taken shape over the centuries in folk medicine have little to do with liquids or ointments that are to be applied to the afflicted area. Rather, most have depended on magical practices.

While warts can bother adults, they seem especially fond of children. And so, were you reared centuries ago, you would have encountered a seemingly endless array of magical cures. The same holds true if you were raised just yesterday in a region or family that still cherishes the folkways of old.

In either case, you might have been told that you need do no more than make the sign of the cross over the wart to be rid of it. Or that you could "throw it away" simply by rubbing it with some pebbles or grains of corn or barley and then tossing them over your shoulder.

If your parents were of a more dramatic turn of mind, they might have had you try the "burial" process in any of its several forms. You could count your warts, put a like number of grains of corn in a box, and bury the box. Or you could massage the wart with a dead apple twig and toss the twig into a field that was about to be plowed under. Or you might rub the wart with your choice of a host of readily available objects— onions, radishes, green walnuts, pickles, raw potatoes, beans, horsehairs, silk threads, chicken feet—and then bury them beneath the eaves of your house. A few swipes of a greasy dishrag across the offending thing, followed by the rag's interment beneath the eaves, would do quite as well. Here, your mother might have thought the rag would serve best if stolen. If she felt a little queasy at the idea of theft, she would have argued that it would work just fine if the rag belonged to the family.

The rubbing could also be done with a strip of bacon rind or raw beef. Each would work best if it were then buried out in the garden. Do we have here magic or a blend of the magical and the practical? I rather suspect the latter. Who wants to run the risk of a bad smell or a hungry animal burrowing about under one's eaves?

If you came from a family with a particularly grim turn of mind, you might have been made to massage the wart with some pebbles, after which you would have tossed them into an open grave. I don't know here whether your family was having you simply bury the wart out of existence or was trying a bit of transference and hoping the wart would be passed on to the unfortunate in the casket. Were transference the tactic, they also could have equipped you with an arsenal of other strategies.

One might have been this venerable and, in Europe and America, still-practiced procedure: rub the wart with a grain of barley that is then fed to a chicken. The disappearance of the grain down the unsuspecting animal's gullet marks the beginning of the wart's disappearance. You can also do well by first making the wart bleed (through rubbing or pricking with a pin), then putting a speck of the blood on the corn, and finally feeding the concoction to a rooster.

Should your family have harbored little compassion for their fellow man, they might have urged you to this stratagem: rub the wart with a few bits of gravel and toss the gravel into the middle of a roadway. The first person who comes strolling or riding past will pick up the wart.

Or consider these heartless stunts. Rub a penny across the wart and toss the coin into the roadway so that someone will pick up the penny and go on his way thinking he has chanced upon a windfall, only to find that he has inherited your wart. Or place your afflicted hand in a bag for a few minutes, then tie the bag shut and leave it in a conspicuous place; the first person curious enough to open it will be gifted with your wart. The same thing can be done by rubbing the wart with a rock and placing the rock in a box, there to wait for the first person who opens the box.

Then there are several tricks that your family might

have had you play on the dead. One calls for you to touch a dead man's hand and then touch your wart; somehow, the deceased will carry the affliction with him into eternity. Another instructs you to stand quietly and respectfully at curbside as a funeral procession passes by. You may be looking appropriately respectful, but what you're really doing is praying that the corpse will be cooperative and take the wart down to the grave, there to be covered over and never able to bother you again.

As odd as these cures are, the one that strikes me as the most fanciful of all has nothing to do with transference. For this one, your family would have you carry a dead cat out to a cemetery at night. Then, holding the deceased by the tail, you'd swing it in a circle above your head three times. But for success, you had to be sure to be standing in the moonlight at the time.

This practice seems to be connected with an old European procedure that involved the lowly mole. It called for the victim to hold a mole that had been smothered to death over his head for a moment. The supposed healing properties in the dead animal were expected to flow downward to the victim's hands. The same cure was used for problems elsewhere in or on the body. In several regions of the United States, a dead mole is still pressed against a wart to effect a cure.

There is at least one cure that involves water. Thanks to Mark Twain, it has found a lasting place in American literature. In *The Adventures of Tom Sawyer*, Twain has his young hero tell Huck Finn of it. According to Tom, you're to go alone into the woods at night, locate a spunk water stump, put your back to it, and, at the hour of midnight, shove your hand into the water housed in the stump and recite:

Barley corn, barley corn, injun-meal shorts,
Spunk water, spunk water, swaller these warts.

Medical dictionaries define the wart as a localized benign hypertrophy (meaning an enlargement or over-growth of an organ resulting from an increase in the size of its cells) of the skin. Its cause is unknown. But no matter. As nonsensical as some of the practices we've mentioned may seem, any one of them can exorcise the wart if one given condition is present. The patient *must* believe that the cure will work. This is why a perfectly useless remedy can do wonders for a wide-eyed child if the adult very solemnly promises that the wart will— no question about it—disappear in five days if dipped in anything from water to chicken soup and then ban-daged over.

In common with many parents, I've seen this work in my own family. When my daughter was five or six, she developed a pretty hefty wart on her left index fin-gertip. Our family doctor, with all due solemnity, in-structed her to dip the afflicted fingertip into Mercurochrome for five nights in a row just before go-ing to bed, after which the wart was to be wrapped in a clean bandage. On the sixth morning it would be gone. And, by God, it was.

I also know of an adult, one of my wife's sisters, who was cured of a large and painful plantar wart in much the same way, except that the doctor now coated the remedy over with a nice veneer of "science." He told the patient that the wart consisted of various bacilli and assured her that they could be smothered out of existence if the wart was heavily bandaged and left undisturbed for a week. He was right.

Possibly the last word on disposing of the hated wart comes from a physician friend. He says, ''There are two ways to kill a wart—by electric needle or hypnotism.''

I had a batch of warts removed from my thumb by electric needle when I was twelve or so and, in the doctor's opinion, a shade too old for any hocus-pocus. I'll take hypnotism—which, in my vocabulary, is another word for magic—any day of the week.

Don't Cross Your Eyes and Other Medical Advice from Mother

Is THERE A ONE OF US who, as children, did not hear some combination—if not every last one—of the following maternal cautions? My guess is that, collectively, they must assuredly rank among the funniest and, at the same time, most deliciously scary of childhood memories:

Don't cross your eyes. They'll stay that way.

Don't make that face. It'll freeze there forever.

Don't stick out your tongue. You'll never get it back in again.

Don't make me yell at you. I'll need the breath when I'm dying.

Don't point. Your finger will fall off. (Or grow warts, according to the recollections of some of my friends.)

* * *

Don't eat for an hour after taking a bath. And don't go swimming for an hour after eating. You'll get cramps.

Don't drink the water in a swimming pool or a dirty pond. And don't put your mouth against the drinking fountain. Your teeth will fall out.

Don't eat so many doughnuts. You'll turn into one.

In my boyhood, this last prohibition held true for eating the ''terrible three''—candy, cake, and cookies. I even remember being told, at about age six, that it was possible for me to turn into an ice-cream cone.

On the other hand, there were these encouragements, most of which were reserved for the dinner table:

Eat your spinach. You'll grow up to be strong like Popeye.

Eat your carrots. Then you'll never have to wear glasses.

Eat your beets. They'll make your cheeks pink.

And this venerable one:

Clean your plate. There are starving children in the world.

The logic here always escaped me. I could never figure out how my eating a full meal would end starvation among the world's unfortunate young. I remember the trouble I got into one night when I suggested that my dinner be put in a box and mailed to Africa or China.

Now to close with two classic "do's":

Always wash your hands before eating.

Always wear clean underwear. You might get hit by a trolley car. (Or, for that matter, any vehicle that your mother would take it into her head to mention.)

CHAPTER THREE

When You Hurt All Over

PAIN: IT IS KNOWN TO US ALL. Depending on its cause, it can be slight, excruciating, an occasional visitor, or a constant companion. To see what folk medicine has done to help us endure or put an end to this universal condition in its assorted forms, we begin with the notorious companion that so inflames and tortures the body's muscles and joints that it was long ago nicknamed "The Great Crippler."

RHEUMATISM

There is no question that rheumatism has plagued humans from our first days on the planet. That it is an age-old affliction has been established by archaeologists who have found its traces in the remains of prehistoric beings.

Nor is there any doubt that rheumatism has struck us wherever we live in the world, and that we have long sought the reasons for its presence and the ways in which it can be prevented or cured. A handful of examples from widely separated regions and eras proves the point:

The aborigines of Australia believe rheumatism to be the nefarious work of an enemy. It comes when he crouches over his intended victim's footprints and presses bits of stone, broken glass, or bone into them. Far eastward, across the Pacific, the Aztecs of Mexico held that Tlaloc, their god of the waters, punished sinners by giving them rheumatic ailments.

Still persisting in some Irish districts and dating back to antiquity is the custom of wearing an iron ring on the fourth finger to prevent or cure rheumatism. In the American Midwest of the 1800s, the skin of a mole—that little creature that was made to battle all types of illness—was worn about the neck as a preventive. The practice continued into our own century.

A number of early societies thought that rheumatic pains could be eased or ended with bee stings. It was common practice for the afflicted to visit beekeepers, who began the treatment with two stings. The number was then gradually increased over a series of visits until the patient reported a lessening of pain. The faith in bee stings as a cure lingers to this day in both Europe and the United States. A similar type of treatment is seen along South America's Orinoco River, where one Indian tribe believes that rheumatism can be cured by allowing a certain species of ants to bite the affected area several times.

Finally, there is no question that both folk and formal medicine have fought the affliction since antiquity with every weapon at their command—medicines; rituals; mechanical and, later, electrical appliances; and magical strategies.

Medicines and Rituals

For centuries, the principal weapons were herbal medications made of a long list of plants. The doctors of ancient times, for instance, had their patients chew the bark of the willow tree, or gave them teas and ointments made from its relative, the black poplar tree, and the meadowsweet plant. They also crushed the leaves of the henbane plant and pressed them against the pained area. The Indian medicine men of northwest America prescribed the drinking of a tea brewed from the needles of either the Douglas or red fir; elsewhere, tribes ground black mustard seeds to a fine powder and mixed them with animal fats to make a paste that was then applied to the inflamed muscles or joints; the Delaware Indians ate the root of the pokeweed plant. For the Europeans of the Middle Ages, oil from the bay tree served as a rheumatic massage.

Modern research has shown that some of these herbal treatments were of genuine value. Those involving the willow and poplar trees and the meadowsweet plant serve as major examples. The bark, leaves, and buds of the willow and black poplar and the flowers of the meadowsweet all yield salicin, a compound of salicylates. The salicylates are salts or esters of salicylic acid, and it is from them that acetylsalicylic acid, the active ingredient in modern aspirin, is synthesized. More about them in a while when we talk about headaches.

Though the willow and its two salicin-bearing companions served as rheumatism fighters for centuries after antiquity (right up to our own century, in fact), most herbal treatments eventually disappeared from western formal medicine, to be replaced by various drugs. Many of those drugs, however, were derived from the herbs, with henbane joining the salicylates as a case in point. It provides us today with the drug atropine, which is used in the treatment of several disorders, among them cardiac arrest.

Though eventually abandoned by formal medicine, many of the old herbal treatments lingered on in folk medicine and are still prescribed today in many areas. For example, there are the several remedies from the American southland that Eliot Wigginton reports in *The Foxfire Book*. For one, you can reduce your rheumatic pains by cooking garlic in your food. For another, try drinking a tea brewed with alfalfa seeds or leaves. Or you might wish to roast a pokeweed root in ashes and, before letting it cool, apply it to the pained area. It is said not only to alleviate the pain but reduce the swelling as well.

It is well that the medication is to be applied externally. The Delaware Indians may have gotten away with eating the pokeweed's root, but for centuries the plant has been notorious for its poisonous effect on humans. For a time in the late 1800s, tinctures of pokeweed were widely sold as rheumatism cures in the eastern United States. Sales understandably came to an abrupt halt when the word got around that the cures hadn't cured at all, but had instead poisoned a number of patients.

As was true in the treatment of all other ills, the herbal remedies for rheumatism were accompanied in antiquity by magical medicines and rituals. The magical medicines—in keeping with the belief that all illness was brought by demons who had then to be expelled—were renowned and feared for their loathsome ingredients (everything, as was said in chapter two, from animal entrails to human excrement). Often, the wiser doctors of the period mixed herbs that they thought or knew from experience to be genuinely helpful into the vile concoctions.

The rituals varied among the cultures. They included rites that had the patients immerse themselves in hot baths or mineral waters (both of which could bring temporary relief); breathe in the smoke from burning plants with sacred, and thus healing, powers; or cleanse themselves of the internal impurities thought responsible for their rheumatic pain by self-flagellation with their hands, whips, or sapling branches. A ritual still observed in Afghanistan requires the patient to beat himself and recite prayers as he walks around a grave.

The use of nauseating medications prevailed for centuries. In the Europe of the Middle Ages, apothecaries (the often benighted forerunners of the modern pharmacist) concocted and sold drugs that were supposed to do good if they were associated with the strange or the frightening, reflecting the grim and superstitious mindset of the era. Representative of their medicines was the bestselling *usnea*, a substance reputedly able to cure any number of debilitating conditions. Usnea is a lichen, but the usnea sold by the apothecaries was a fuzz scraped from the head of a criminal who had been hanged. It was widely admired by physicians—even the most enlightened—for the next few centuries and remained in use as an internal medicine until sometime in the early 1800s.

Appliance Cures

Appliance cures are those that were reputed to heal through the use of some magical, mechanical, or electrical gadget. Usnea provides an example of one such cure for rheumatism and other painful conditions. In this instance, usnea itself was not employed but rather the rope with which the criminal had been hanged. To the people of the Middle Ages, the rope was endowed with magical powers because it had been responsible for a man's death. And so the hangmen and charlatans of the day turned a profit at the hands of a superstitious public by cutting the rope into as many pieces as possible, with each piece then being sold to some rheumatic, arthritic, or gouty victim on the premise that it would heal when massaged against the troubled body part.

Actually, trust in the magical powers of a hangman's rope was nothing new at the time. It can be traced as far back as the day when the Roman naturalist Pliny the Elder (A.D. 23–79) wrote in his *Natural History* that the rope could be used to cure a headache: all one had to do was to bind the pained temples with it. Pliny's *Natural History* is a massive treatise on the ancient sciences and, though branded today as containing little of genuine scientific merit, was respected throughout antiquity, up until the Middle Ages.

Pliny's belief was gradually extended to include a variety of illnesses. Also, the ropes that had been used in suicides were increasingly thought to have magical powers. In the eighteenth and nineteenth centuries, such illnesses as ague, fevers, and rheumatism were thought to be curable simply by carrying a piece of the hangman's rope on one's person. A strip of suicide rope, when worn about the neck, supposedly made a person immune to accidents and fits. Somewhere along the line, another fancy took shape—that a length of execution or suicide rope was a pretty lucky thing to keep around the house.

The popularity of the usnea rope as a rheumatism cure in the Middle Ages was matched by the use of other appliances in later times. One of the most famous of the lot was invented by possibly the most infamous medical charlatan of all time—Italian-born Count Alessandro Cagliostro. He reaped a fortune from the wealthy of the 1700s with his "rheumatism chair," which, he claimed, provided freedom from pain if the user simply made a habit of sitting in the contraption. Cagliostro then went on to foist his "childbirth bed" on the gullible wealthy, guaranteeing that the woman who stretched herself out on it at the time of delivery would be blessed with an easy time of things. Probably, however, Cagliostro reaped his greatest profits from the magical concoctions he devised and peddled throughout Europe—elixirs that kept one forever young, potions that increased one's amatory powers, and medicines that miraculously made ugly women beautiful.

Still another widely used appliance cure appeared on the scene at the close of the eighteenth century, when Dr. Elisha Perkins of the United States patented his "tractors" for treating various ailments, especially, his advertisements held, rheumatism, arthritis, pleurisy, and gout. Perkins has been branded a charlatan by some historians, while others argue that he was quite sincere in his belief that his tractors really worked. The Connecticut doctor was honest enough to admit openly that the only painful ailment his appliances were helpless to end was the hangover headache.

The Perkins tractors were simply two metallic rods that were placed against the skin. Each measured about three inches long, was flat along one side and rounded along the other, and was pointed at one end and rounded at the other. Perkins touted them as being constructed of gold, silver, copper, platinum, and zinc. Because he manufactured the things in an oven in his home, these elements strike many as being a little too complicated for him to have handled. The suspicion is that the tractors were made of a mixture of brass and iron.

Whatever the case, they were placed on the affected area and held there until the skin turned red, or they were drawn downward towards the hands or legs (an upward movement was said to run the risk of pushing the malady and its pain deeper into the body). According to the doctor, the metals in the tractors created an electrical current that eased the pain and effected a cure.

The "Perkinese tractors," as they were called, became highly popular in the United States (George Washington was among their admirers) and abroad during the early 1800s, in great part because people of the day were fascinated with the idea of electricity. The doctor patented his invention just a short time after Italy's Luigi Galvani had announced that he'd seen a frog's legs move when under electrical influence, namely when touched by different metals. Some years earlier, Benjamin Franklin had amazed everyone when his kite experiment proved that lightning is electricity. Helping matters along at the dawn of the new century was Italian scientist Alessandro Volta's invention, the "voltaic pile"—the grandfather of the modern electric battery.

Possibly the most recent of the appliance cures was the work of "General" Jacob S. Coxey (1854–1951), the patent-medicine manufacturer and the leader of the Depression-era march of veterans on Washington D.C.

to demand payment of their bonuses for service in World War I. In 1945, when he was ninety years old and abed with a severe rheumatism attack, Coxey happened to read about Galvani's work and was inspired to invent his "electric heels," which, he happily announced after testing them, had succeeded in reducing his pain. What he did was insert a small zinc plate into the heel of one shoe, and a copper plate into the other. Coxey said they generated an electric current that provided the needed relief. He immediately christened them Cox-E-Lax and put them on the market with his other patent medicines.

Folk Magic

As far as pure fascination is concerned, though they do make interesting reading, the appliance cures can't hold a candle to the magical treatments that folk medicine has given us. Of all such treatments, perhaps the most fascinating are those involving transference. They range from the exotic to the cruel to the very simple. Consider:

From French Canada comes this odd ploy for transferring rheumatism to a tree. As described by Luc Lacourciere in *American Folk Medicine: A Symposium*, it calls for the sufferer to go alone into a wooded area, pick any tree that strikes his fancy, and dig its root out with his left hand. Then he is to place the root between his teeth and, while holding it there, say: "Rheumatism, I leave you here and will take you back when I pass this way again." He completes the ritual by reburying the root with his left hand. Now that he has passed the rheumatism into the tree, he employs the most obvious of strategems. He makes sure that he never goes near the tree again.

Next, there is the old Irish tactic that is a variation of a heartless wart cure. Rheumatism victims are to hold the hand of a corpse and, as its casket is carried out the front door on its way to cemetery, shout "Take my pain with you!"

Far less complicated are the folk treatments that call for the sufferer to wear an everyday object, the potato being a prime choice. In Europe and America, the potato has long been regarded as both a cure and a preventive if carried about daily (usually in a pocket on the pained side of the body) until it rots and needs to be replaced. There are two folk theories on how the potato does this double duty. The first holds that it cures through transference by drawing the rheumatism out of the patient. The second maintains that it serves as a preventive by passing its unknown but nevertheless potent anti-rheumatic properties into the body.

Running a close second to the potato—and likewise carried on one's person—are the buckeye and the nutmeg seed. The buckeye is the large nut-like seed of the European horse-chestnut tree and its American relative, the buckeye tree. For centuries, Europeans grew the horse-chestnut tree for decoration and did not learn of the medicinal potential in its seed until they saw the Indians of the New World using the seed as a cure for rheumatism and other ills, among them hemorrhoids. Word of what they saw was sent back home, and the horse chestnut's seed was put to new work.

The carrying of the nutmeg seed is an old European custom. In certain British districts, the wearing of nutmeg is reputed to cure rheumatism, lumbago, gout, and boils. (As practiced in one English district, the method by which the nutmeg cures boils is especially interesting and works on the same principle as a number of wart cures. To begin with, the nutmeg must be given to the sufferer by a member of the opposite sex. Then, as the victim carries it about, he or she is to nibble on it now and again. By the time the nutmeg is fully consumed, the boils will have vanished.)

Now, beginning with one of the basic colors in the spectrum, here are some magical cures in which transference may or may not play a part. Is it present in some that work by absorption as the potato does? Or do they work by some other kind of inexplicable magic?

Just as the color blue is thought to play a role in curing the common cold, so has red long served as a folk preventive and cure for rheumatism. For example, in the 1800s some British ladies believed that wearing red garters would hold the ailment at bay. As late as our own century, many of the people of Wales believed that a patch of red flannel safeguarded one not only from rheumatism but from fever and smallpox as well. Still persisting in both Europe and the United States is the belief that a red string worn about the neck will keep rheumatism away.

But why is red trusted as an effective preventive and cure? It is because, in folklore and legend, the color has long symbolized magic, and so was early thought to be imbued with a mysterious power to heal numerous ills. The Welsh faith in red flannel as a safeguard against smallpox may date back to the fourteenth century, when a physician announced that he had cured an English prince of the dread disease by placing red and scarlet cloths on the boy's pustules. In later centuries, red cloths and ribbons were brought to bear against nosebleeds and sore throats, as they are yet today.

Iron is also still used as preventive both in the United States and abroad. The Irish are not alone in believing that the wearing of a finger ring of iron serves well to prevent and cure. An old English preventive—with a dash of magic tossed in for good measure—calls for the potential victim to adorn his hand with a ring made of three nails taken from three coffins located in three different churchyards.

The faith in iron can be traced back to antiquity. Rome's Pliny the Elder, again in his *Natural History*, claimed that white-hot iron, after being immersed in water, served as a useful medicine in a variety of ills. He also remarked that rust, usually secured by scraping old nails, helped in the treatment of wounds by drawing the skin together and that, when placed in liniments, it was effective against swellings and gout.

Pliny's admiration for iron is reflected in such still-practiced remedies as wearing a nail from a horseshoe or coffin—or taking one or the other to bed with you. In some regions, the faith in iron has been extended to other metals. An old European and American remedy, for instance, calls for rheumatics to sleep with a piece of steel under their pillow. A pair of scissors is a convenient choice here.

A Miscellany

The folk remedies we've mentioned thus far, while being among the most widely used, are actually but a few in comparison with the total available for thwarting rheumatism. Here, to round things out and presented without comment, is a sampling from that total, beginning with an assortment of aged cures that you will hear advised even today:

Tie a salt mackerel to your feet.

Spice your food with garlic.

Wrap the pained area in a dried eel skin.

Rub Spanish pepper into your fingernails. This is a popular treatment in parts of Indonesia.

If you've the courage for it (or are desperate enough), you might try this antique Welsh remedy: stand naked in a hole in a graveyard, have your friends cover you up to the neck with dirt, and then remain a prisoner there for two hours. Repeat the process nine times.

And what of preventives? Some answers:

Take a cat or dog to bed with you and transfer the problem to the poor thing while you sleep. In some regions of the United States, especially in the southwest, the dog is preferred, with the Mexican hairless being a particular favorite.

If the above idea holds little or no appeal, sleep with glass knobs under your bedposts.

Wear rattlesnake rattles in your hat. Or hang one of the rattles on a string and wear it around your neck. Or fashion a headband of rattlesnake skin.

Wear the eyetooth of a pig.

Look for turtle doves nesting near your home. In a number of rural areas of the United States, they are thought to keep rheumatism away.

ARTHRITIS AND GOUT

Arthritis and gout are relatives of rheumatism. As such, their treatments through the ages have often matched those for rheumatism. The early beekeepers, for instance, not only loosed their charges on rheumatics but on arthritics and the gouty as well. The willow, poplar, and meadowsweet approaches were likewise used. So were suicide and execution ropes, the disgusting usnea, and Dr. Perkins's tractors.

Early on, however, formal medicine apparently began to think that some medicinals did better with one or the other of these complaints rather than with all three equally. For example, although salves and medications made from the autumn crocus were brought to bear against the trio, the plant was directed principally against gout. The Egyptians are thought to have eased gouty pains with it more than four thousand years ago. The Greeks, Romans, and the Arab doctors of the Byzantine Empire are known definitely to have turned to it for the same purpose. The plant worked well because it yields the alkaloid colchinine, which is today administered intravenously or by capsule to combat gout and is known to stop oncoming attacks and prevent the condition from recurring.

The folk treatments that remain today for arthritis and gout are many. Some are aimed at one or the other, while others are identical to those for rheumatism. Among the former are these:

> For arthritis, drink a tea made from the leaves or seeds of alfalfa. This remedy is much admired in the United States Appalachians and the South. The faith in alfalfa may date back to the early Arabs, who looked on it as such an excellent staple that they named it *al-fashfash*, meaning "best fodder." They thought of it as a fine food for themselves and fed it to their horses for strength and speed.

> For gout, there's this old-time cure from eastern Europe: place a mole's tooth (ah, once again, the poor and much-beleaguered mole) in a sack and wear it about your neck.

And what of the preventives and cures that are identical to those for rheumatism? The wearing of a red flannel patch will keep gout away. You can cure or prevent arthritis by going about with either of those trusty weapons—the potato or the buckeye—in your pocket. The same can be done by carrying a metal device, this time a magnet; it will draw the arthritis out of the body.

HEADACHE

The headache is, in part, responsible for one of the world's earliest surgeries—trepanning, or trephining. The surgery, which is still performed today, involves boring into and removing sections of the skull. It dates back some 25,000 years to the Stone Age, and is thought to have been employed to free the patient of the demons of headache or insanity.

That the surgery was widely performed is evident in the fact that archaeologists have unearthed several hundred prehistoric skulls, all of them bearing the roundish holes of trepanning, in such widely separated areas as Europe (England, France, Portugal), Canada, Mexico, and South America (Argentina and Peru). The largest number—more than two hundred—have been discovered in France.

When the skulls were first studied, it was thought that the trepanning had been performed on corpses, probably to obtain "magical" bits of bone that could be worn as amulets. But a closer inspection revealed a staggering fact: there was new bone growth surrounding many of the holes. The operation—done with crude flint tools, the only surgical instruments available at the time—had been performed on living patients and had been performed so expertly that many had survived the ordeal, with the amount of new growth indicating that they had lived on for anywhere from several months to several years. One South American collection of four hundred skulls showed evidence of two hundred and fifty recoveries, while one skull from another group indicated that the patient had survived no fewer than five trepannings.

Out the window went the idea that the operation had been performed to obtain the material for charms and amulets, replaced by the theory that the world's first trepannings were intended to ease headache and insanity.

Today, 25,000 years later, aspirin is the world's most widely used painkiller, inexpensively relieving not only headache but usually all pain except gastrointestinal distress. It was invented in 1853 by chemist Charles Frederick von Gerhardt when he made acetylsalicylic acid while working in a laboratory at France's University of Montpellier. Since the acid is a synthetic form of the salicylates, his invention is connected to a treatment perhaps almost as old as trepanning. When faced with headachy patients, doctors in antiquity recommended medications from those distinguished foes of rheumatism and its related conditions—the salicylate-rich willow and black poplar trees and the meadowsweet plant.

Extracts from the threesome served as headache remedies until the dawn of our own century—almost fifty years after von Gerhardt created aspirin. The reason: he failed to test his new drug extensively and made the mistake of thinking that it worked no better than the salicylate extracts. It was not until 1893 that a chemist with Germany's Farbenfabriken Bayer AG drug company, in a desperate search to find some relief for his father's arthritis, turned to acetylsalicylic acid and found, to his delight, that it did wonders for his parent's agonizing and crippling condition. By the close of the 1800s, the Bayer company was producing the new drug from the meadowsweet plant, whose botanical name is *Spiraea ulmaria*, and marketing it under the brand name Aspirin. The company devised the name by taking the *a* from acetyl- and the *spir* from *Spiraea*. The *in* was tacked on because it had long served as a suffix for a variety of commercial medicines.

Despite the availability of the reliable and inexpensive aspirin, the people in many a European and American rural area still chew the bark of the willow or turn to a string of other age-old cures when hit with a headache. Should you be similarly bothered while among them, you'll likely be greeted with the following suggestions, some of which you'll recognize as doing duty with other complaints:

Bind your head with the rope which has been used to hang someone, either by execution or suicide.

Drink a little soda water if your headache is caused by indigestion.

Place two matches on the forehead in the form of a cross.

Sleep with a pair of scissors under your pillow.

Place a toad on your head. When the toad dies, your headache will be gone.

Apply crushed peppermint leaves to the forehead. The leaves should be freshly picked.

Find a person who has had a mole die in his hand. Have him place that hand against your forehead.

Now suppose that a friend or a loved one has a headache. You can do the victim a good turn simply by gently rubbing his or her scalp. The headache will be transferred to you. But not to worry. The pain will now be less severe and will soon pass.

Finally, if you'd like to avoid headaches altogether, you should gather up all the clippings after you've had a haircut and bury them under a rock. Headaches will never bother you again.

This practice is an outgrowth of the centuries-old superstitious fear that strands of your hair, if lost or carelessly thrown away, are bound to cause you trouble. A witch might pick them up and use them to bring you under her spell. An enemy might use them to do you harm. A bird might build its nest of them and condemn you to a lifetime of headaches. Worse, if a magpie lines its nest with any of your lost discarded strands, you're sure to die within a year and a day.

But why this dread that your discarded or lost hair will cause you troubles that could include death? It seems to stem from an old belief that God counts all the hairs on our heads and that we are to appear whole on Judgment Day and so are expected to have them all in hand at that time. Out of this belief stemmed such customs as never burning cut hair but always burying or carefully storing it away instead.

But, since human views are varied and contradictory, this belief is balanced by ones quite the opposite. In some English districts, it is considered bad luck for you to save your fallen or clipped hair. The same holds true for parents who save the clipped hair of their children. Both parents and children are sure to meet early deaths.

COLLECTIBLES

Odd Beliefs

IF YOU'RE NOT simply browsing through this book, and you have not turned to this page at random but have read all that has gone before, you know that folk medicine has more than its fair share of odd beliefs and treatments. Some of the oddest, however, have nothing to do with the topics discussed in the various chapters. And so, to get them on the record, we begin with a sampling of the beliefs among their number. We'll get to the odd treatments after the next chapter.

Always cover your mouth when you yawn. This will keep evil spirits from entering your body.

If you wish always to have a good memory, never read the epitaphs on headstones.

New England

Never comb your hair after the sun has gone down. It will make you forgetful.

southern United States

Never whip a child with the branch of a green broom plant. The youngster will stop growing.

England

Avoid drinking coffee at five o'clock. Otherwise, you will die.

southern United States

If you kiss your elbow, You will turn into a member of the opposite sex.

Never pick up flowers found lying in a roadway or elsewhere. Rather, always heed the following warnings:

Pick up a flower,
Pick up sorrow.

Pick up a flower,
Pick up sickness.

CHAPTER FOUR

Love for Some,
Lust for Others

ONE OF THE OLDEST and most familiar of saws holds that "Love makes the world go round." It's an axiom that folk medicine has taken seriously since antiquity, surrounding the matter of romance with an abundance of potions, charms, aphrodisiacs, and fertility practices. Many in each of these categories got their start in early formal medicine and religious ritual.

LOVE POTIONS AND CHARMS

Plants, animal parts, and human parts—all served as ingredients in the potions and charms that were devised in centuries past to trigger love in a person who was cool to or unaware of one's ardor. Potions were liquids or foods that you usually slipped to your "victim" on the sly. Charms were amulets of one sort or another that you wore to attract another or secreted somewhere on the body of your unsuspecting beloved.

Plants

Possibly the most famous and popular of the plants used in ancient love potions was the mandrake. A native of the Mediterranean region, poisonous in all its

74

parts, and a member of the nightshade family, the plant has a history that dates back to and beyond Old Testament times. Among the ancients who knew of it were the Assyrians, Hebrews, Babylonians, Egyptians, Greeks, Romans, and Chinese. The Greeks associated it with their goddess of love, Aphrodite, and frequently referred to her by the name Mandragoris. They also associated the plant with Circe, the legendary sorceress who played a seductive and evil role in the travels of Odysseus and his men. When they paused to explore her island home, Aeaea, while sailing home from the battle at Troy, she first enamored them and then turned them into swine with a magic potion. The potion was variously believed to have been an infusion of mandrake.

(Only Odysseus, who is credited with the idea for the Trojan Horse, managed to escape their fate. He protected himself with an herb that easily matched mandrake's fame throughout antiquity and then through the subsequent centuries to this day. It was, however, honored as medicinal rather than as a love plant—and, on learning its name, you'll understand why. Odysseus knew it as *moly*. We call it garlic.)

Wherever the mandrake was grown, it was held in deep awe because it is a plant whose root is bifurcated and thus bears an eerie resemblance to the human form, with each root stem once commonly called a "thighe." In affairs of the heart, the plant served two purposes. It supposedly not only prompted a reciprocal love on the part of someone when insinuated into a potion but also served as an aphrodisiac, reputedly triggering fiery sexual desires in its users. The Greeks hid it in wine or vinegar when intending it as an aphrodisiac.

Though its fame has always rested principally in its reputation as a love plant, the mandrake was widely used for other purposes. European superstition for centuries held that, worn somewhere on the body, it would render the wearer invisible. It was also said to cure all diseases, hold evil spirits at bay, improve one's marksmanship, and point the way to buried treasure. Because the plant has mild narcotic properties, it was employed in formal medicine as a surgical anesthetic from antiquity through the Middle Ages, at which time physicians began to abandon it in favor of other plants, such as the poppy with its opium content, that were recognized as having greater narcotic powers.

As was to be expected, a number of superstitions grew up about this seemingly magical plant. The historian-statesman-author Flavius Josephus (c. A.D. 37–100), wrote that it shrank from anyone who came near it and that it was fatal to anyone who touched it. According to a widely-held European belief, the plant grew only under a gallows and was given life by the juices flowing from the body of a hanged man (another example of the grip that the victim of a hanging had on the ancient imagination). The victim had to be what was known as a "pure" criminal, that is, one who had been a miscreant all his life. Another belief had it that the plant, because of its human shape, screamed when pulled from the ground and brought a terrible consequence that Shakespeare's Juliet expressed:

And shrieks like mandrake torn out of the earth,
That living mortals, hearing them, run mad.

Romeo and Juliet
Act IV, Scene III

Anyone who heard that shriek would not only be driven mad, but would also die in agony.

The mandrake's promise of death at the touch prompted Flavius Josephus to recommend a safe method for collecting it, a system that persisted through the centuries, as long as madness followed by death was prophesied for anyone who heard its scream. Were you to gather the plant, Josephus advised that you carefully dig a hole around it until only a portion of its root still remained embedded in the ground. Then you were to tie a dog to the root, walk to a safe distance, and summon the animal. The dog would tear the root free and would either die as he obeyed your command, or soon fall ill with a fatal disease. In time, variations of this strategy took shape. One was to starve a dog for three days and then, on tying the animal in place, drop some food a short distance away. But how were you to protect yourself from being driven insane and dying when the uprooted plant loosed its screech? By covering your ears with your hands. Or shouting. Or blowing a horn. Or pulling any stunt that drowned out that lethal sound.

The mandrake was for centuries also known as the "love apple." The term was likewise applied to the apple itself because its many seeds prompted the idea that it could induce fertility. Today, the apple still serves as a love charm in a number of United States superstitions. For one, if you were a smitten young woman who was raised in the South, you might have been told that, should you but go about with an apple tucked under your arm and then eat it when it has grown warm, you will make the young man of your choice love you. The apple is also a source of amorous trickery in Newfoundland. There, according to an old superstition, you'll win the object of your affections if you punch a number of pinholes in an apple, carry it about for a time, and then hand it to your beloved.

The tomato was also dubbed the love apple long ago, but only as the result of an etymological mixup. At the time when it was imported into Europe from Africa, the tomato was known as the "apple of the Moors," with the mix-up occurring when it made its way to France. There, the people confused the word *Moro* (for Moor) with their word for love, *amour*, and gave the plant an undeserved reputation as an instigator of romance. When the Spanish encountered the tomato plant in South America, they decided it assuredly contained the same properties as its European relative, called it the love apple, and quickly credited it with being a powerful erotic medicine. The idea that the New World branch of the tomato family was an aphrodisiac persisted until recent times.

A United States plant with a root similar to that of the mandrake is the mayapple. With the exception of its fruit, it is poisonous in all its parts. The mayapple is widely known as the American mandrake, but is not related to the Mediterranean plant. Though the Indians failed to think of the mayapple as a love plant, they did make it perform several medical tasks—as a laxative, a means of aborting pregnancies, and a cure for such disparate ailments as warts and intestinal worms. The Algonquians brewed it as a spring tonic. Its poisonous contents led a number of tribes to use it as a vehicle for suicide.

Though the mandrake was one of the most—if not *the* most—popular and trusted of the love plants, it was far from being the only one put to use. In Europe, the oil of the caraway plant went into love potions because of the ancient superstition that anything containing caraway oil was safe from theft. Thus, a young man or woman might secrete the oil in a drink in the conviction that the recipient would never be stolen away by another. The Welsh mistook the black and white bryony plants for the mandrake and credited them with its supposed love powers; they then went a step further and envisioned the two as being of separate sexes, calling the black bryony the *man*drake, and the white variety the *woman*drake. In western America, Indian women covertly fed the California poppy to husbands or lovers whose ardor did not strike them as being up to snuff. Insulted and annoyed, the men retaliated by outlawing the tactic: any woman caught trying it was expelled from the tribe.

Animal Parts

An imaginative but misplaced logic can be seen in the choice of certain of the animal parts that went into the early love potions and charms. According to *Funk and Wagnall's Standard Dictionary of Folklore, Mythology, and Legend*, animal testicles were popular choices for infusion into potions by many primitive peoples, with the Australian aborigines, for instance, using those of the kangaroo, and the American Indians those of the beaver. The Creoles of Louisiana favored a love recipe (still used today) that called for the hearts of hummingbirds to be roasted and ground into a powder that was then sprinkled on the object of one's desire.

Some animals, however, seemed illogical choices, with one looming as especially frightening and bizarre. There was a time in central Europe when a young woman, frustrated by a reluctant beau, would add a few drops of a bat's blood to his beer in the hope of changing his ways and driving him into her arms. At the time, as had been the case for centuries, the bat was suffering a terrible reputation among the Europeans. For them, in part because of its ugliness and in part because of its ability to fly in the dark, the little creature was associated with witches, ghosts, and death. In Scotland, the glimpse of a bat rising and then dipping back to earth was a sign that the hour had arrived when witches would be at their full powers. To those in southern England, a bat flying in through an open window signified an approaching death in the family.

However, the dislike and fear of the bat was not shared by all Europeans. There were those who looked on the bat as a lucky animal and prophesied misfortune for anyone who killed it. The Hessians of Germany thought that the gambler who sat at a card table with the creature's heart tied to his sleeve with a red string would emerge from the play a winner (once more, the faith in the color red shows itself). The heart and the red string may be linked to the ancient idea that the bat's blood gave the animal its uncanny ability to fly in the dark. In turn, the fancy that the bat's blood could bring luck at cards might have triggered the equally fanciful idea that it could bless the ardent but ignored young lover.

Incidentally, the connection between the bat and love was not limited to Europe. Far across the world, an aboriginal tribe in Australia's New South Wales looked on the animal as a symbol of love.

As for charms, *Funk and Wagnall's Standard Dictionary of Folklore, Mythology, and Legend* reports an early African-American use of what seems another un-likely animal—the lowly frog, so disliked, in part be-cause of the superstition that it gave warts to anyone who touched it. But the choice of at least one of the animal's parts had a certain logic to it. The charm took shape when the lovelorn imprisoned a live frog on an anthill and left it there until the ants had eaten away all its flesh. Of the bones that remained, two—one heart-shaped and the other hook-shaped—were then re-moved. The lovelorn kept the former, but quietly at-tached the latter to the beloved's clothing.

A similar charm was mentioned in the 1849 book, *Narrative of the Life Adventures of Henry Bibb: An American Slave Written by Himself.* Bibb wrote of how a witch doctor told him that he could make any girl of his choice fall in love with him if he simply scratched some part of her body with a bone that had been taken from a bullfrog and then dried. The witch doctor claimed that the charm would work no matter what the woman was doing at the time, no matter with whom she was currently enamored, and no matter whether or not she was a stranger to Bibb. The trusting Bibb did as counseled—with unhappy results, when he flicked the bone across the back of the neck of a comely pas-serby. All that his amorous experimentation won was a yowl of pain and an infuriated stare. But what else could he expect as a stranger who had, without warning, etched a long furrow in the woman's skin?

Human Parts

Transference played—as it still does—the chief role in the use of human parts in love potions and charms. The idea here was to pass some part of oneself on to the reluctant or unaware target of your affections. This was done surreptitiously, and supposedly transferred to him or her one's own feelings.

The list of transference items was long. It included anything that could be easily secreted in a potion or charm. For example, you might transform a broth or a cooling drink into a potion by infusing it with a few drops of blood—not a bat's this time, but your own. The same could be done with an infusion of your perspiration or saliva. A sprinkle of bathwater in the broth or drink was the choice of many young European and American women at one time.

As for charms, had you been raised in the Europe or the America of another day, you would have early learned that a few drops of your saliva or bathwater would work romantic wonders if dotted on a handkerchief that you then presented to your beloved as a gift. You would have also learned, however, that the most popular charms intended for hiding on the loved one's person were strands of hair, pins, fingernail parings, and tiny swatches cut from your clothing. My great-grandmother believed that a snippet of cloth cut from an item of a young lady's intimate wear worked best of all.

It was common practice for you or the local witch doctor or witch to recite a magic incantation over the potion or charm before it was put to work. (A special word must be said here on behalf of the witch. While feared in many areas, the witch somehow was at the same time regarded with respect and affection. In many villages where formal medical care was not at hand— or not trusted—it was she to whom the people turned for the magic concoctions that cured their frightening and bewildering ills. And it was her help that you would seek when you required a love potion of special strength.)

Believers in transference have long said that it can also work in reverse, and that you will be loved in return if you take something belonging to your beloved. A venerable superstition in the American South advises that a young man need do no more than pull a hair from the head of the one he desires. The process is somewhat more complicated for the young woman. To achieve the hoped-for result, she must not only pull a hair from the man of her dreams but must then also bury it alongside one of her own. Another southern superstition holds that you can win an ardor that matches the depth and fidelity of your own by secreting a lock of your beloved's hair in your hat. It will insure that he or she will never be tempted by another.

Potions and Charms: A Miscellany

Not all charms and potions were administered secretly. Nor were they invariably prepared by the one whose feelings were going unappreciated. For example, two lovers, especially if facing a separation for a time, were apt to mix the juice of pansy petals into a potion. They did so because tradition held that the colors of the petals—white, purple, and yellow—symbolized loving thoughts, memories, and souvenirs. The potion was said to soothe the lovers' hearts, making the separation bearable and insuring that neither one need worry about the danger of "out of sight, out of mind." It was this intimate use of the pansy that gave it the alternate name by which it is still known—heartease.

It was also common practice for lovers to exchange

charms as tokens of their affection. Among the items most frequently traded were locks of hair, pieces of clothing, drops of blood, and, as is still done to signify engagements and marriages, rings. Quite often, the woman wove her hair into a bracelet for presentation to her beloved as a symbol of her enduring affection and fidelity; the man's acceptance of the gift constituted his pledge of unwavering faithfulness to her. In Australia, the women of the Arunta tribe, a people living now much as they did in the Stone Age, braid their hair into necklaces to be worn by the men of their choice.

APHRODISIACS

Named for the Greek goddess of love, aphrodisiacs are foods that, when ingested, are alleged to trigger intense sexual desires. As with the love potions, the centuries from antiquity onward saw a wide variety of foods— plants and animals alike—ingested for the sexual stimulation they promised. Some were chosen because of their suggestive shapes. Among them, of course, was the mandrake, due to its uncanny resemblance to the human form. But ranking alongside it due to their shapes were the fish and the vanilla plant, the former because it reminded people of the penis, and the latter because of the resemblance of its pod to the vagina. It is from the Spanish word for vagina—*vaina*—that the name of the plant is derived.

Competing with the above two in the love arena were a string of other plants and animals. The asparagus, the banana, the carrot (dating back to the time when Pliny the Elder wrote that it contained aphrodisiacal properties), and the eel—all resembling the phallus—were popular options. So was the oyster, as it still is today, because when on the half shell, it resembles the female's outer genitalia.

The choice of a food as an aphrodisiac also depended on character traits that the ancients noted in an animal or a plant. The fish, for example, was a favorite not only because of its phallic shape. The ancients, as was said in an earlier chapter, were also impressed by the sexual connotation of its ability to swim through—penetrate—water, and by the fact that it lays a prodigious number of eggs. There is also the fact that it contains phosphorus, which, according to our forebears, had been seen to arouse certain animals when ingested in heavy doses. The encyclopedic work *Man, Myth, and Magic* reports the case of a drake that, after accidentally drinking phosphorus, so lusted after a gathering of ducks that he died of exhaustion.

(As an aside, it's interesting to note that the fish, like the bat, has long been burdened with a dual reputation. While many of our forebears considered it a symbol of fertility, others looked on it as representing sexual indifference. As a result, centuries later, we are well acquainted with the derisive expression *cold fish*, which means either a person of frosty nature or one of meager sexual impulses. The latter meaning was more commonly used in bygone days and stemmed from the fact that some fish are able to produce their young without mating.)

The reasons why other plants and animals were chosen are difficult to pinpoint and understand, because there is little or nothing in them that is sexually suggestive, either in their physical shapes or their character traits. One of the lot is the ocean shrimp. Its reputation seems to rest on a short passage in the writings of Giovanni Casanova (1725–1798), the Venetian author and adventurer famous (or infamous) for his seemingly endless seductions. He wrote that he credited his sexual prowess to a supper eaten by his mother on the eve of his birth—a meal that consisted of a bowl of spiced shrimps.

Nor can any sexual connotation be detected in the mistletoe, lavender, or southernwood plants. Yet the druids of England ate the mistletoe to increase their potency, and for centuries the parasitic plant was considered a fertility "drug" throughout Europe. The reasons why mistletoe earned this reputation are so old that they have been lost in the mists of time. One possibility is that the plant was once thought to take its life from bird droppings that landed on tree branches—a thought that stems from the ancient idea that dung is a sacred and life-giving substance. Whatever the reason upon which mistletoe's fame in romance may rest, its association with love and sexual play remains with us today at Christmastime. The tradition of kissing under a sprig of the plant dates back at least to the Lupercalia, an annual Roman fertility festival. More about it later.

The lavender plant, most likely because of its delicate aroma, was considered an aphrodisiac by the Europeans of the Middle Ages. Actually, they felt it served two quite contrary functions: on the one hand, it aroused the passions; on the other, if its water was sprinkled on the head of a young woman, she was destined to remain chaste.

Southernwood, a plant native to Spain and Italy that is now grown throughout the eastern United States, once enjoyed such a widespread reputation as an aphrodisiac that it came to be known variously as the lad's love, maid's ruin, and lover's plant, and found its way into both love potions and perfumes. In addition, it was thought to cause beards to grow swiftly, with the upshot being that young men who wished to look virile and older than their actual years daily massaged their faces with its leaves.

Southernwood was long made to do medical as well as erotic duty. It was put to use for antiseptic, diuretic, and worming purposes. There was a validity to these services. Southernwood contains the oil *absinthol*, which is recognized today as an effective agent against intestinal worms, insects, and certain germs. One of the plant's more unusual medical uses saw its lemon-scented leaves fashioned into nosegays that were carried into courtrooms by attorneys, judges, jurors, and spectators, there to be sniffed as a safeguard against a mysterious malady known as jail fever.

It is also impossible to find anything sexually suggestive in the notorious beetle—the *Cantharis vesicatoria*—that long ago gave us what is still reputed to be one of the most potent of all the aphrodisiacs—Spanish fly. It's a good guess that the beetle won its fame through its ability to irritate the genito-urinary tract. The ancients might have been—or thought themselves to have been—sexually aroused by this action, but we today recognize it as being dangerous. As was said earlier, it can induce cramps and internal bleeding and, when ingested in even small doses, can—and does—kill.

Do any of these reputed aphrodisiacs actually stimulate sexual desire? The answer appears to be no. Modern research into the various aphrodisiacs, while not extensive, suggests that most do not contain sufficient quantities of substances, such as phosphorus, that are known to have an effect on the genito-urinary tract, with the notable exception of Spanish fly, whose actions on the tract may be sexually arousing but are far too dangerous for personal experimentation. Further, the fact that many were chosen for their suggestive shapes and character traits indicates that their effect on their users, if any, was triggered by auto-suggestion.

FERTILITY PRACTICES

Since so many plants and animals were made to perform multiple duties in folk medicine, it should come as no surprise that the mandrake and the fish also played a role in the fertility practices of old.

Early on, the mandrake was prescribed to end barrenness in a woman. *Genesis* (XXX:14–16) tells of how Jacob's wives, Rachel and Leah (the former barren and the latter beyond the age of child-bearing), used the mandrakes gathered by Leah's son to become pregnant by their shared husband. The trust in the mandrake as a fertility food persisted through the centuries, with British poet John Donne (1572–1631) writing:

> Goe and catche a falling starre,
> Get with child a mandrake roote.

As for the fish, a number of ancient peoples—among them the Egyptians, Assyrians, Babylonians, Phoenicians, Greeks, Romans, and Chinese—looked on it as a fertility symbol, again partly because of its phallic shape, but perhaps most of all because of its talent for laying an extraordinary number of eggs. The fish as a fertility symbol was responsible for a variety of odd beliefs. Consider:

The Carib Indians of the Caribbean region said that the fish was always young and that any man who lived on a fish diet would likewise always remain young, with his sexual and reproductive powers undiminished.

Or take these stories reported by folklorist Eric Maple in *Man, Myth, and Magic*:

The people of Medieval Europe burned fish as part of their fertility practices and rites. The odor of the burning fish, so they believed, would drive away evil spirits hostile to love and procreation. Behind the practice may have been a tale written two centuries before Christ. The *Book of Tobit*, one of the writings in the Apocrypha, contains an incident in which a burning fish put to flight a spirit that interfered with love.

Presented to virgins in India, Samoa, and Brazil were gifts of fish to induce pregnancy. The practice continues to this day, and is accompanied by tales of women actually having been fertilized by the gifts.

The husband of a childless wife in the South Pacific was instructed to travel to the "Childless Sea" on the coast of Java. There, he was to take a fish from the water and eat it. His wife would then stand a better chance of bearing him a child.

The natives of Greenland long believed that the eating of certain fish would produce an unforgettable result—pregnancy in both men and women.

But what of the other fertility practices? Because its many seeds suggested an ability to fertilize, the apple was the choice of Etruscan women, who eagerly devoured it after it had been blessed by their priests. When the first sea-swallow egg was found on the South Pacific's Easter Island, where birds held a prominent place in legend, it was filled with fibrous tapa and employed as a fertility charm. The coconut has long been esteemed in India as one of the most sacred of foods, and was early given by priests to women experiencing difficulty in conceiving. An old but still used southern United States folk cure for barrenness calls for the woman to eat cooked dog meat, a treatment perhaps grounded in the fact that some early societies looked on the dog as a fertility symbol.

Many a childless Englishwoman of another time believed that, if she walked naked in her garden on Midsummer Day (June 24) and picked the flowers of the St.-John's-wort, she would be pregnant before the next Midsummer Day. The plant, thought to house magic properties that not only induced fertility but also fended off evil spirits and ghosts, was said to attain its greatest power around Midsummer Day. Much of that power, so legend held, came from the plant's yellow flowers. In color symbolization, yellow is scorned as representing cowardice and treachery, but denotes magical properties when seen in a blossom. Sprinkled against the wort's yellow background as the flower matures are red dots. These symbolize the blood of St. John the Baptist, for whom the plant is named.

The majority of fertility practices seem to have been intended for women. But there were some for men as well. For instance, the Amazon male thought he could increase the size of his penis (and, as a result, his potency) by beating the organ with the fruit of the *aninga*, an aquatic plant that resembles the phallic-shaped banana. Perhaps most widely used by troubled men is what may well be the greatest of all the fertility symbols, because it is the vehicle in which so much beginning life is carried—the egg. In a Serbian region, according to *Man, Myth, and Magic*, the man who is fretting about his virility applies, as his ancestors did, fried eggs to his testicles. The Moroccan male with the same problem starts his mornings for forty days by eating an egg yolk.

Fertility practices intended for both men and women—in fact, for entire communities—were presented in ritual form in virtually all ancient societies. They could either be presented on their own in the form of dances and accompanying ceremonies or as part of festivals. The festivals were usually held in observance of special days or times of the year.

Among the most famous of the lot historically was Rome's Lupercalia festival. Held in mid-February, it took place at the Lupercal, the spot where the twins Romulus and Remus, the legendary founders of the city, had been suckled by a she-wolf after being abandoned when their mother, the Vestal Virgin Rhea Silvia, was condemned to death for conceiving them. The festivity was highlighted by the sacrifice of several goats, after which the priests in charge of the affair dressed themselves in the skins of the sacrificed animals, fashioned whips from what remained of the skins, and topped things off by running through the streets and lashing anyone they chanced upon. Any woman wishing to conceive eagerly awaited their arrival, for, when struck by the whips, she was said to be rendered fertile and to be fated to bear her future child with ease.

The goat's central role in the festival came of the fact that he ranked as a major fertility symbol for the Romans (and a number of other peoples as well). Actually, the animal was viewed in two different ways in antiquity. His stubbornness and agility caused the ancients to see him as a symbol of persistence and of the admirable ability to overcome obstacles, but they also early associated him with Satan and evil, primarily because of his insatiable appetites and disgusting odor. From there, it was but an imaginative step to brand him as a figure of lust and lechery, a concept that is yet echoed in our day in such commonplace expressions as *old goat* and *old billy goat*, both referring to aging, lecherous men. The Greeks took the concept so seriously that they developed the lusty and ever-on-the-make god Pan, with his human torso and goat's head, loins, arms, and hooves. The Romans, master imitators rather than innovators when it came to concocting deities, borrowed Pan from the Greeks and gave him a name of their own, Faunus.

It may be titillating to think of these fertility rituals, the Lupercalia among them, as being orgiastic affairs. But the truth of the matter is that the vast majority, in both advanced and primitive societies (especially the latter), were not intended for mindless sexual pleasure. Though they often featured phallic symbols and highly suggestive dances (involving kissing and the meeting of abdomens), they were primarily aimed at propagating the race or tribe and increasing the yield of its life-sustaining foods, plants, and animals. The intent to propagate the race can be clearly seen in a ritual dance that is mentioned in Japanese mythology. Accompanied by shouts of the dancer and the striking of a bucket, the dance was performed to catch the ear of the sun-goddess Amaterasu, who, terrified by the strange actions of her brother, had fled to a cave in the heavens and had left the world in darkness. Once her attention was caught by the dance, it was hoped that she would be lured down to earth, bringing with her the return of light and life.

The desire to increase the yield of crops is evident in the old European festival held on Maundy Thursday or, as it was once known, Green Thursday. Farmers would devote part of the day to coating their plows with eggs in the hope of insuring a bountiful harvest.

Finally, to see what was done to increase the animal population, we can travel back to the hunters of prehistory. There remains much evidence that Paleolithic man practiced what seems to have been fertility magic to insure an ample supply of game. The magic took the form of drawings and sculptures of animals, always depicted in couples, the implication in such depictions being inescapable. Among the sculptures that have come down through the centuries to us, sheltered in French caves, are those representing bison, reindeer, and a bull and its mate. The drawings also include one of a graceful doe and her faun.

COLLECTIBLES

Odd Treatments

If you have ringworm, you can be rid of it by finding a girl between ages twelve and sixteen and having her rub the toe of her right foot in a circle around the infected area for a minute.

United States Ozarks

Remember the stitch in your side that you used to get as a child after running a distance? Had you only known, you could have eased it by rubbing it with a flat stone. You then had to spit on the stone and return it to the very spot where you found it.

If you're bothered by nightmares, you can be rid of them with a simple tactic at bedtime. Take a few sniffs of the socks or stockings you've worn that day.

New England

A child who is suffering impetigo can be cured by having a left-handed person hold the youngster in front of a cupboard door that is then opened and closed a magical three times.

French Louisiana

If a child falls ill with mumps, rub the swollen area with wood chipped from a pigsty.

Should you be burned or scalded, seek out someone who has licked the head, torso, feet, legs, and tail of a lizard. His or her tongue has the power to heal both burns and scalds.

Ireland

For my money, the first prize for the oddest of all folk treatments goes to one in the book *Grannie's Remedies*. It's for tapeworm, and I'm willing to bet that you'll wonder how anyone ever managed to take it seriously. But author Mai Thomas writes that her grandmother claimed it was a common remedy at one time. To effect a cure, you're to:

Have the patient go without eating for three days. Then, with the patient in the room, cook a large steak. Hold it in front of the patient's mouth. Out will jump the ravenous tapeworm.

Well, what do you think? My first reaction was to wonder if ''Grannie'' had trouble keeping a straight face whenever she mentioned it. But who can tell when it comes to odd treatments?

CHAPTER FIVE

'Til Death Do Us Part: Marriage and Babies

THE MARRIAGE CEREMONY is surrounded by folk beliefs and practices. Most—such as the admonitions that the bride wear "something borrowed, something blue" to the altar and that she and her groom always return home by a route different from the one that they took to the church—have to do with insuring good fortune for the couple. Since good fortune invariably includes good health, it can be said that the majority have a tenuous connection with specific health and medical matters. Only a handful can claim a sturdier linkage:

The bride and groom are to kneel at the altar in the same moment. Should they ignore or forget this injunction, the first to kneel will be the first to die. The same holds true for the first to fall asleep on the wedding night.

The bride must save a piece of the wedding cake for the christening of her first child. She will be barren if she fails to do so.

From the moment she is married, a woman must never drop, remove, or lose her wedding ring. Otherwise, bad luck is certain to follow, including the death of her husband.

As for the ring itself, it is worn on the fourth finger of the left hand because of the ancient medical belief that a sensitive nerve extends from that finger to the heart.

Matters change dramatically, however, when the young bride becomes pregnant. She is then immersed in a sea of folk beliefs, customs, and practices meant to promote her comfort and safeguard her health and that of her child. Ranging from the practical to the fanciful, they cover all aspects of her life—her pregnancy, her delivery, her behavior after delivery, and the care of her newborn child.

A CHILD IS ON THE WAY

For many a woman of yesteryear, especially the farm woman, childbearing was virtually an unending task. Large families in rural areas were the rule of the day for any of several reasons. Often, the children were needed to work the land with the parents. Often, the parents believed that they were performing as God desired and intended they should in producing large broods. And there was also the fact that some couples proudly regarded their large family as a sign of the husband's manliness and the wife's fertility.

Let us drop back a century-and-a-half and say that you are a woman of the land, perhaps somewhere in Europe, perhaps somewhere in the young United States. It is probable that you do not look on birthing, despite its discomforts and inconveniences, as a terrible burden. Rather, more often with anticipation than resignation, you accept it as a God-given duty in which pride as a woman is to be taken. The young city lady might affect a delicate constitution and the pallid complexion and swooning spells that go with it. But not you—and not any of your sisters of the soil. You and your kind are giving agricultural history the tradition of women who work the farm—milking the cows, swilling the pigs, churning the butter, and helping behind the plow—right up to the moment of birth, and then, on delivering and placing the newcomer safely in a crib, return to the day's chores. (In fairness, however, it must be said that authors Madge E. Pickard and R. Carlyle Buley, in their *The Midwest Pioneer: His Ills, Cures, & Doctors*, point out that such instances, while there is a sufficient number of them on record to establish the tradition, were not actually in the majority. Childbirth held obvious dangers, and country women met it with due caution.)

As a newlywed of the mid-1800s, you are well aware that the experienced wives around you, excited and amused, are eagerly anticipating the first signs of pregnancy—the sudden onset of morning sickness, your odd turns of appetite, your growing interest in child-raising. Should you fail to become pregnant soon enough to satisfy their expectations, they may advise you to pick some parsley or plant some of your own. Either way, they say, it will increase your chances of bearing a child. (But things may become a bit confusing for you here, because some of the wives may come from regions where the reverse is held to be true—that any traffic with parsley inhibits conception.)

If they're of a teasing bent and you're quite young

and naive, the wives might suggest that you put your faith in another strategy:

Place a lump of sugar outside your window or on its sill. The stork will come for it and bring a baby.

They may not realize it, but the good ladies are voicing a European superstition of unknown but ancient origin. All that can be said is that many European myths, especially in the central and northern regions of the continent, hold that the stork fetches unborn infants from caves, rocky places, wells, ponds, springs, and marshes, and brings them to waiting families. It is interesting to note that the legends concern a water bird and, for the most part, involve watery collection points; is this coincidence or is there an imaginative link here with the fact that the unborn child is housed in a protective fluid? Some of the legends also speak of babies being brought by the swan, another water bird.

But once the good wives have determined that you are indeed, in the pretty phrasing of the day, "in a family way," their teasing ends. They now happily descend on you with an unwritten almanac of practical, down-to-earth folk predictions and advice.

The fact that medical testing to determine the sex of an unborn child is as at this time yet undreamed-of does not stop them from predicting whether your little one will be a boy or a girl. All that is needed, they proudly contend, is an alert and knowing feminine eye. If they see you carrying the child straight to your front, you're certain to have a boy. If the abdomen is spread out to your sides, count on a girl. (My grandmother was either a remarkably lucky gambler or had a genuine knack for this type of prognostication. She rarely missed in correctly forecasting the sex of any soon-to-arrive youngster by looking at how it was being carried.)

Your friends may also attempt another test. They'll attach your wedding ring to one of your hairs or to a length of string or silken thread and suspend it over your abdomen. The ring will soon move (perhaps unconsciously helped by an excited hand), and this action will let everyone know the sex of your baby. There may, however, be some disagreement among the women in their interpretation of the action. For some, a rise and fall of the ring indicates a girl, while a circular movement promises a boy. For others, the circular motion has a prophecy all its own: if clockwise, it betokens a girl; if counter-clockwise, a boy. Should you be reluctant to remove your wedding ring for the experiment (remember the bad luck promised by the removal), you can turn to such substitutes as another ring, a bead, or a darning or crochet needle.

Many of the wives' predictions are sure to concern the influences that your prenatal behavior will exert on the child. For one, you'll likely be told that if you read the Bible in its entirety during your time, your child will grow up to be a minister. For another, if you listen to music, play an instrument, or sing while pregnant, you can pretty well count on the youngster being musical. If you maintain a happy disposition throughout your nine months, you will produce a happy child. Quite simply, what is in play here is transference in another of its varied forms.

Transference is also on the mind of the neighbor who cautions that upsetting experiences and the foods that you find yourself craving can affect the child adversely.

This is to be expected, because the child is a part of you and can be expected to react just as your body reacts. More often than not, they will mark the newcomer with one kind of skin blemish or another. Bearing witness to this grim view are the following accounts of experiences and beliefs that Austin Fife lists in *American Folk Medicine: A Symposium*. Collected in the mid- and late-1900s by the folklorist, his wife, and students in the folklore classes at Utah State University, the accounts were gathered principally from people living in Utah and the surrounding regions, with Fife remarking that a number of the beliefs made their way westward from Europe:

One man credited a gray spot on his body to the fact that his mother was frightened by a mouse during pregnancy.

A woman said that a friend was frightened by a snake while carrying. Her child was born with the outline of a snake circling its head. The reptile's head was located between the youngster's eyes.

One interviewee cautioned that a pregnant woman must never look at a fire. Otherwise, her baby's face will be stained with a birthmark that resembles red burns.

Nor, according to other interviewees, is she to eat or pick strawberries. They will cause the child to be born with a birthmark resembling the fruit. The same applies to the picking of raspberries. And she should never open an umbrella indoors, lest her child's head be covered with a birthmark.

From still other interviewees: A pregnant woman who eats a potato with a spoiled spot on it will give birth to a deformed child. But the child of a woman who eats carrots will be blessed with fine eyesight.

As for advice on medical care, the wives around you have their fair share of remedies for the physical discomforts that accompany pregnancy. A chief target will be that almost daily trial—morning sickness. Its remedies vary from locale to locale. If you live in the American South or Southwest, you will probably be urged to sip a glass of water laced with a dash of baking soda; it will reduce your queasiness by neutralizing the acids in your stomach. If you happen to be a New Englander, a teaspoonful of apple-cider vinegar in the water will be recommended. If your home is in any of several United States regions, you'll likely be told that the eating of starch will provide a sense of comfort throughout your time.

The wives are also certain to caution you never to stoop over your laundry basket and then reach up to the clothesline; it's a sure way to wrap the umbilical cord around the baby's neck. You're also bound to hear that two practices should be routinely observed to insure an easy—or easier—delivery. First, make a habit of drinking raspberry-leaf tea. Second, always sleep with an axe under the bed; this one stems from the ancient belief that the axe is magically able to cut the pain of all illnesses and or injuries. Then, to help matters along, the axe is to be left under the bed during delivery. (Some of the folk strategies for insuring an easy delivery are quite as old as the faith in the axe, among them the custom of the women in ancient Mexico to wear necklaces fashioned from the shells of the sea snail. The belief was that the woman's child would then slip from her as easily as does the snail from its shell.)

THE BABY ARRIVES

When your labor begins, you become the central figure in an experience that is cloaked in practices that may well date back to prehistory. In themselves they are interesting, but they become amazing when we remember that they did not originate in just a few neighboring societies. Rather, they were observed by cultures, both advanced and primitive, throughout the ancient world. Though many of the societies presumably had no communication with the others—and, indeed, presumably no idea that the others even existed—they all still managed to develop unmistakably similar birth customs and outlooks. Either there was more global communication at the time than we realize or, as is perhaps more likely, we have here a splendid example of the commonality of the human imagination.

To see these practices still at work in your time and society, we begin with a most commonplace one. On entering labor, you are secluded from all except those who will assist in your delivery; among those banished from your presence is your husband. Obviously, your seclusion is meant to provide a needed and desired privacy. But there is more to it than that. At play also is an echo of the awe and fear with which blood—especially menstrual and parturient blood—was viewed by the most ancient of our ancestors. Recognized as a basic life force, blood was said to be especially potent during menstruation and at the time of delivery. At birth, it carried and attracted life spirits that threatened terrible dangers of contamination for all concerned, including the child. And so the woman went into seclusion not only to satisfy her own need for privacy, but to safeguard the people nearby from being harmed by those spirits. Thus began the tradition of dispatching the father, not just to keep him from getting underfoot in what was seen as women's work, but in great part to protect him. The other men nearby were likewise sent scurrying. And *scurrying* is the right word here. The women made no bones about wanting to be rid of the males.

In some locales—Africa, Borneo, and South America among them—there was yet another reason for exiling the husband. He was sent off to observe a number of practices meant to help protect his child from certain dangers. One such practice was *couvade*, which got its start in societies that were changing from matrilineal to patrilineal and was first used to help the father lay claim to his rights in the child. Once the birth was accomplished, couvade called for him to abstain from drink and specified foods and to avoid hunting and other kinds of work. Behind this was the idea that, since the child was as much a part of the father as the mother, these activities could injure the delicate newborn. There was also the notion that, since each was a part of the other, both the child and father were weakened by the ordeal of birth and needed to rest. In some regions, the father went through a lying-in period and conjured up the same pains that his wife endured. Depending on the society, the period of couvade could last from a few days to several weeks. Often, it continued until the mother had undergone postnatal purification rites, which usually took place a week or so after the child's arrival.

It should be pointed out that not every ancient society banished the husband and his fellow villagers or tribesmen from the scene of the birth. In some cultures, all the male relatives were expected to be on hand, and the husband was expected to help in the delivery or take charge as the midwife.

But back now to your own delivery and the seclusion that marks its start. Depending on where you live, you might be required to retire to a special place—perhaps the family barn, as is done in Russia's Smolensk region; perhaps, as is the custom in India and Africa, your mother's home or a spot behind it; or, as is the tradition among some North American tribes, a secret place in the forest. But, living as you do in a rural European or American region of 150 years ago, you will probably seek out your bedroom—or whatever corner your bed occupies if your home happens to be a hut or a cabin without such a nicety, there to be curtained off from view.

The birth itself may be supervised by a medical man. But since you are a country woman, the chances are that you will be attended by a midwife. There may be no doctor within miles. Or you may prefer the midwife's ministrations; after all, it was a midwife who served your mother and her mother. There may be an added reason for your preference; it may be that, in some instinctive and primeval recess of your being, you are harking back to the old belief that all men must be separated from the birthing scene for their safety.

For whatever reason she is chosen, your trust in the midwife is usually well placed. She and her kind have spent a lifetime supervising deliveries and, in many cases, are as expert at their work as a medical doctor. Theirs is a calling that dates back to antiquity, when they were known and accepted in such widely separated nations as Greece (where their duties were formally outlined), India, and China. At times, their practices were benighted and cruel, as in Europe during the Middle Ages, but this is because the European medicine of that era was itself, for reasons we'll see in a moment, benighted and cruel. They are widely respected by the women of your day, and their successors will continue to be respected in rural communities throughout the world for years to come and will still be practicing their art as the twenty-first century dawns, with many admired by professional medicine and many working to improve the obstetrical care and facilities in their localities and offering practical counsel on birth control.

Expert though your midwife is, she is nevertheless subject to the superstitions of her time and place. And so she may begin by taking several "magical" steps to insure your easy delivery and the safety of your child. She may hurry through the house, unlocking all its doors as she goes, convinced that this ceremonial journey will somehow "unlock" you as well. If she was raised in any of numerous European nations—Germany and Hungary among them—she may well take another step and stuff the keyholes with cloth. Her intention here is to keep changelings from endangering the coming infant. Depending on the beliefs of the given country, changelings are the deformed and moronic children of underground dwarfs, demons, fairies, or witches.

They are said to steal into the birthing room and take the place of healthy, attractive infants when the infants are left unguarded or are awaiting the safety that comes with baptism. (Europe does not hold the franchise on the belief in changelings. They are also feared in various other regions, with two distant examples being the Philippines and the South Pacific.)

As part of her preliminary care, the midwife can be expected to check that you obeyed the counsel to keep an axe under the bed throughout your pregnancy; if it's there, she will leave it alone; if not, she will fetch one to take care of things. She may use a piece of flint as a substitute if she wishes; it is believed by some peoples to work quite as well. She may also place a chunk of iron or an implement made of iron in your bed, this not to ease your delivery but rather to protect your child from being replaced by the changelings or stolen by the other spirits that accompany a birth. If either of you comes from Ireland, a pair of your husband's trousers will be gently draped about your neck to reduce the coming pain, apparently be transferring it to one of his possessions.

Should yours be a difficult delivery, the midwife will turn to the technique called "quilling." She will insert snuff into your nostrils to make you sneeze and thus assist the passage of the child. The technique may strike you as cruel and trying when you are in the throes of labor, but it is as nothing when compared to the procedures used by other cultures to hasten a reluctant birth.

Some American Indian tribes placed the woman in an open field and then sent horsemen charging down on her, only to swing away at the last possible second. One early Greek procedure was to lift the mother repeatedly from her bed and drop her back down again. Another saw her strapped to a narrow bed that was then set on end and bounced. In time, due in great part to the teachings of Hippocrates (460–377 B.C.), Greece was given a far kinder and wiser medicine—a medicine that was a genuine science—and abandoned these devices. But they reappeared in the Europe of the Middle Ages when, as physician Howard W. Haggard writes in *Devils, Drugs, and Doctors*, the prevailing Christian outlook was that pregnancy resulted from a carnal sin that could be erased only through suffering great pain. Out of this view came the ugliest of childbirth practices. One was the attempted use of intrauterine tubes through which baptismal water could be poured so that the soul of the child hopelessly trapped in the womb could be saved before mother and child were left to die. Another was the use of a long-abandoned Greek invention—the childbirth chair; one glance at it can leave no doubt as to how the child would enter the world: the contrivance was nothing more than a toilet seat. Such brutal treatments as these, along with the absence of any prudent hygienic measures whatsoever, took the lives of countless women and infants. They finally began to disappear in the sixteenth and seventeenth centuries, when the intelligence previously exhibited by the Greeks emerged in European medical circles, and the view that childbirth was the outcome of an evil was gradually replaced by the concept that it was instead a God-given privilege.

THE NEW BABY

As soon as your baby is born—let's say a girl to be named Jane after your mother—the midwife will take steps to safeguard the new arrival from the dangers of the contaminating birth spirits. She may massage Jane with a protective oil. Since your home is somewhere in Europe or the United States, she will unfailingly dress the little one in a gown that is startlingly long. This is done to disguise Jane as an adult in the hopes that any spirit interested in stealing an infant will overlook her. As an added precaution against theft, she may hide a small piece of iron—as she did in your bed—or a pinch of salt somewhere in the gown. She may well regard the salt as a safeguard against both theft and illness and as a beginning contribution to Jane's character; ever since antiquity, salt has been admired as an efficient healer and has served as a symbol of incorruptibility and perpetuity. Almost without doubt, the midwife will dress Jane from the feet up, certain that it's bad luck to bring a child's first clothing down over the head. Should she see tiny ears thrusting outward, she will undoubtedly cloak Jane's head in a snug-fitting, helmet-like muslin cap to press them back to their appropriate and attractive places.

If you and the midwife are English or Irish, Jane's first gowns may be those meant for a boy, for this, by some magic, will insure that she will one day prove appealing to men. You may also think it a good idea to dress your future male children in girl's clothing. In so doing, you will make them safe from theft by boy-seeking spirits. (In some Irish districts, it was common practice to dress boys as girls until they were twelve to fourteen years old.)

Once she has met Jane's immediate needs, the midwife will attend to the placenta and the umbilical cord. In the folk beliefs found in both advanced and primitive societies worldwide, these are magic objects that are variously thought to contain the child's soul-substance or guardian spirit, with some cultures looking on them as the infant's twin or double. Thus, they are inseparable from Jane's soul, her character, her destiny, and her eventual death. The midwife knows that the way in which they are now tended can well determine the fortune, good or bad, that the future years will send Jane's way. And so they must be safeguarded at all costs. The placenta, for instance, must not be thrown away or lost, lest it be found by an evil spirit or eaten by an animal. Should the latter occur, all the creature's ugly aspects will be passed to Jane. Rather, it should be buried or preserved in some manner determined by local custom and belief. It is the tradition in many societies, both advanced and primitive, to bury the placenta beneath the eaves of the house, this to engender in the child a loyalty to the home.

As for the umbilical cord, it can be tended to in a number of different ways. Should the midwife come from the area around Berlin, Germany—or have been reared in its traditions—she may present the cord to your husband with the admonition that he zealously preserve it for all time to come; for so long as it is preserved, so will Jane live and be free of sickness. But, should the midwife come from some other German region, she may wrap the cord in linen and then, after a time, prick it to pieces with a sharp instrument, this to turn Jane into an expert seamstress. Should you later have a boy, she will then hack the cord to pieces with the idea of making a fine workman of the child.

Attention will also be given to the caul if Jane is born with this membrane covering her head or face. It will be carefully preserved because, echoing a view that has been held since antiquity, you and the midwife know it to be an infallible sign of a life of good fortune for the newcomer. Part of that good fortune is the fact that Jane will always have seamen as ready customers for its purchase at a handsome price; for centuries, they have treasured it as a safeguard against shipwreck and drowning. In some areas, along with being lucky, Jane will be said to be blessed with the talent to tell fortunes and the ability not only to see ghosts and spirits but to talk with them as well. But, though the caul is a happy sign for Jane, the midwife will nevertheless examine it closely for the medical information that it reveals. If firm to the touch, it indicates that Jane is in good health. However, regardless of its rosy promise, it indicates illness if limp.

The caul, should she be born with one, is but one sign of what lies ahead for Jane. Her birth prompts an array of superstitious practices that are intended first to help you divine her coming years, and second to help keep her safe from the dangers that life holds for the infant. For your first glimpse into the future, you might look at Jane's hands and hair. If her now-tiny fingers give promise of being long and slender, she will be a pianist or artist (but you can count on some neighborhood biddy insisting that they're also the sign of a pickpocket). And God forbid that Jane should be born with two thumbs on one hand; they're not only unsightly, but also the sure mark of a thief. As for her hair, you'll be happy if it's of a dark shade, especially if you're a New Englander; up there, light hair tokens poor eyesight.

Or you may prefer to look to the future with this all-too-familiar rhyme, hoping that, based on the day of the week on which Jane arrived, it promises happiness for her:

Monday's child is fair of face,
Tuesday's child is full of grace,
Wednesday's child is full of woe,
Thursday's child has far to go,
Friday's child is loving and giving,
And Saturday's child must work for a living,
But the child that is born on the Sabbath Day,
Is bonny and merry and glad and gay.

In a variation of the verse, the final lines read:

Born on a Sunday, never shall want;
So there's the week and the on't.

The rhyme, which is thought to be British in origin, will undoubtedly trouble you deeply if Jane is a Wednesday child. So will a version heard in the American South: Wednesday's child is sour and sad. But take heart. In New England, this child is loving and giving. If that isn't enough to ease your misgivings, you can always place your faith in the following variation. It will be best to pass it by, though, if Jane is a Thursday or Saturday child:

Born on Monday, you'll have good health,
Born on Tuesday, will make wealth,
Born on Wednesday, born to power,
Born on Thursday, many losses to endure,
Born on Friday, loving and kind,
Saturday's child lags far behind,
Sunday's child has a contented mind.

All the versions agree that the Sunday child is the most fortunate of the lot—for an obvious reason. To the Christian mind, the child whom God saw fit to bring into this life on His day—the Sabbath—could not help but be especially blessed. Speaking most clearly of this belief is the final line in a variation heard in the American South:

To heaven its steps shall tend away.

Now, with the verse read (and hopefully promising a fine future for the child) what must you to do to keep Jane safe from harm? Here is what you'll undoubtedly hear from all the wives who saw you through your pregnancy:

You're to take the greatest care that Jane never sees herself in a mirror before she is nine months old. Otherwise, her life will be cut short. In certain American and European areas, a premature look in a mirror will cause rickets in the child. (Both these beliefs may be linked to the fear of contaminating birth spirits, with the idea perhaps being that the evil things are present in the mirror, in Jane's reflection, or are able to strike at her through her reflection. It may also be that the whole idea is to prevent Jane from becoming vain.)

Death will likewise be Jane's fate if you cut her hair before her first birthday. (Again, a safeguard against evil birth spirits, or a plot to thwart vanity?)

You must not pare her fingernails before the close of her ninth week of life. A paring before then will condemn her to a life of scratching for a living. You will also risk turning her into a thief.

When Jane is too old for her crib and begins to make her way about the floor, you must act quickly should you see her crawling between the legs of a chair or table. You must turn her around immediately so that she crawls back out along her path of entry. She will stop growing if you fail to do so. The same quick action is required if her exploring takes her under a bed.

There are also things you can do to insure Jane's future happiness. One of the most charming—and this one shows no fear of sinful vanity—calls for you to wash her face with baptismal water, for then she will be beautiful all her life.

You will know of and follow a series of other child-protection customs if you live in certain British districts. Iona Opie and Moira Tatum have listed these in their encyclopedic work, *A Dictionary of Superstitions*:

When Jane is first brought to you, her father, or any other family member, she is to be given a gift, usually bread, salt, or eggs (and often all three), to insure her a life of happiness and good fortune. The same gifts are expected of friends when they come to visit the newcomer or are visited by her for the first time.

You are to make certain that anyone who visits Jane or enters the house for any reason following her birth is given some spirits to drink before departing. Your omission here or the refusal of the guest to accept the drink are unthinkable breaches of conduct that will result in the child's early death. If you live in Yorkshire, it is the custom to offer wine, pepper cakes, and cheese to all who enter your home from the moment of an infant's birth to the day of baptism. The guests unfailingly accept them as a gesture of wishing the new arrival happiness and good fortune.

When the moment comes for Jane to leave your room for the first time, you must insist that she be carried upstairs before ever being taken downstairs. This practice guarantees that she will rise in life. But what if your bedroom is located on the top floor of your home? You can solve the problem by stepping up on a chair, a stool, or a low chest as you carry the child to the door. The task can also be performed by your husband, a nursemaid, or a friend or relative. On the other hand, if your home has but a single story, the person carrying the child is to step up on a chair or ascend a two-step riser that has been fashioned for the occasion.

Despite all your initial efforts to shield Jane from life's misfortunes, she is bound in the next months to suffer a variety of common infant complaints. The wives around you will be ready, as always, with their kind and helpful advice. Here, for example, is what they'll suggest for two complaints that no newborn has ever managed to avoid:

Colic

Massage Jane's stomach gently with castor oil that has been slightly warmed.

Feed her breast milk with a drop of kerosene in it.

To avoid the colic altogether, make sure that no one rocks her cradle when it is empty.

Teething

When Jane is teething, gently rub her gums with red coral or whiskey.

If you live among the French in Louisiana, you'll want to have Jane sip a tea made by boiling the leaves of the lizard's-tail plant.

Let her chew on a small piece of bacon rind. It will provide comfort and have the added benefit of teaching her to chew. But always tie a length of string to the rind. Then, should Jane swallow it, you can quickly come to the rescue.

Starting right at her birth, you can safeguard Jane from toothache for her entire lifetime with a simple but admittedly distasteful stratagem. Routinely massage her gums with the brain of a rabbit during her first six months. A rattle from a rattlesnake will also prove effective.

Should she be born with a birthmark, three remedies are at your disposal. The first two are quite as distasteful as the one above, and so you will likely choose the third:

Massage the birthmark for three successive days with the head of a live eel. Use a different eel each day. Then tie the three heads together and bury them under a stone beneath the eaves.

Rub it with the hand of a corpse.

Massage the birthmark with a fresh egg every morning for seven days in a row. A fresh egg is to be used daily. After the final treatment, bury the lot under your doorstep.

As Jane grows older, she will be subject to the same illnesses and injuries that can trouble any member of your household. A sometimes seemingly endless number of home remedies are available to you. They are all contained in your family's "folk-medicine chest," which is now to have a chapter of its own.

COLLECTIBLES

Some Thoughts on Death

Death is the poor man's physician.

Ireland

Death defies the doctor.

O death, where is thy sting?
O grave, where is thy victory?

Genesis

Nothing can happen more beautiful than death.

Starting from Paumanok
Walt Whitman (1819–1892)

Nothing is certain but death and taxes.

This is the last of earth. I am content.

John Quincy Adams (1767–1848)

Count no man happy until he dies.

Daughters of Troy
Euripides (484–406 B.C.)

Call no man happy till he is dead.

Agamemnon
Aeschylus (525–456 B.C.)

Fear of death is worse than death itself.

Diogenes the Cynic, when a little before his death he
fell into a slumber, and his physician rousing him out
of it asked him whether anything ailed him, wisely
answered, "Nothing, sir; only one brother anticipates
the other—Sleep before Death."

Consolation to Apollonius
Plutarch (A.D. 46–120)

Nothing in his life
Became him like leaving it; he died
As one that has been studied in his death
to throw away the dearest things he owned
As 'twere a careless trifle.

Macbeth
William Shakespeare (1564–1616)

CHAPTER SIX

'Til Death Do Us Part:
The Folk-Medicine Chest

It would be a mistake to think of the folk-medicine chest as merely a cabinet or a trunk located somewhere in the home. For many a family, it indeed was and still is. But it was also, as it is yet, a body of lore that was imprinted in the memory or recorded in the family Bible for passage from generation to generation. What has come down to us is a compendium of practical and fanciful methods for the cure and prevention of every ailment and accident—from the most commonplace and potentially harmless to the most dangerous—that can befall a human being.

We've already talked of what can be done for many of these complaints, among them rheumatism, the headache, the common cold, and the ignominious wart. Now, what help does the folk-medicine chest hold for still others? Taking the ailments in alphabetical order, here are some answers.

AGUE

Ague is today defined as malarial fever or any other severe symptom of malarial origin. But the term has long been a confusing one, this because malaria is marked by chills, fever, and uncontrollable shaking. Consequently, any illness that was not actually malaria but was marked by its symptoms and could not be linked to some other known malady, such as flu, was for centuries called ague—or, as it was otherwise whispered with dread, "the fever."

Historical records show malaria to be one of mankind's oldest known infections. In the fifth century B.C., Hippocrates studied the disease, divided its fever into definite types on the basis of when it raged (daily, every other day, or every fourth day). A half-century after the great physician's death, malaria, with an assist from alcoholism, took the life of Alexander the Great (356–323 B.C.) during a stay at Babylon.

Malaria is a global disease that strikes rural and tropical areas in particular. Its fondness of these regions, with their heavy mosquito populations, eventually gave nineteenth-century scientists the key that unlocked the mystery of its cause—transmission by the anopheline mosquito. An effective remedy, however, had been on the scene for centuries prior to turning of that key. Sometime in the early 1600s, Jesuit missionaries in Peru saw the Inca Indians treating the quakings, fevers, and chills of various diseases with the bark and roots of a certain plant. In time, after the plant had been brought to Europe, it was christened with the name by which it is known today, cinchona. The name is in honor of the Countess of Chinchon, the wife of the Spanish Viceroy of Peru, who was long credited with having introduced the plant into Europe.

It was all a mistake. The Countess was said to have brought the plant to Europe on a voyage home to Spain in the late 1630s, but research has established that she died of ague or an ague-like disease while en route, and that the cinchona was not in her luggage at the time. The facts of the matter appear to be that, sometime earlier in the decade, Jesuit priests carried the plant across the Atlantic. Once in Europe, it quickly became a prized adversary of ague. The reason why its roots and bark worked so effectively remained unknown for centuries, but was eventually revealed to be their quinine content. Quinine served as the world's most effective malaria fighter until recently, when it was replaced by synthetic drugs. Quinine itself remains on the market today in hair preparations, suntan lotions, and over-the-counter drugs. It is the source of several other medicinal drugs, among them quinidine, which, like digitalis, is employed to regulate the heartbeat.

But suppose that you and your family lived in the time before cinchona made its way out of Peru. Or that, once the plant had reached the outside world, you were without the means to obtain it. How did you fight the dread ague with the weapons in your folk-medicine chest?

Various medications derived from the local plant life could be brought to bear. For one, you might concoct a tea made of boneset. The plant was not used simply for relief from flu, as was mentioned in chapter one, but was directed against fevers of all types because it was thought to induce a heavy, fever-breaking perspiration. Its widespread use led to the names by which it is still commonly known—agueweed and feverwort.

You could call on the bark and roots of the sassafras tree for a medication that the early Spanish explorers learned of from the Indians in what later became the state of Florida. The Indians brewed a tea of the two and used it as a health tonic, a curative for rheumatism, and, because it, too, was thought to induce heavy perspiration, a treatment for fevers of all types. When the word of its alleged powers reached Europe, sassafras won such a reputation as a fever fighter that it was was christened the ague tree. In short order, because it was also admired as a general cure-all, sassafras became a major export to Europe from the early American colonies, second only to tobacco.

Though sassafras was long regarded as a cure-all, modern research has established only that it serves effectively as a diuretic and carminative (an agent that reduces intestinal and stomach gas). It provided the flavoring in root beer and chewing gum until the 1960s, when the United States Food and Drug Administration announced that the oil in its roots yields a potentially carcinogenic compound. Since then, sassafras has not been employed commercially in the United States.

Far outnumbering the plant medications available to you in olden times—and not unexpectedly because of the lingering ancient fascination with the mysterious—were magical treatments. They were to be found the world over, and the late Sir James George Frazer, in his multivolumed *The Golden Bough*, mentions several that have been long practiced in Europe. Two of their number entail transference. They instruct you to pass your chills, fever, and shivering to a tree:

An Italian remedy has you begin by tying a thread around your left wrist at night. Early the next morning, you are to tie the thread to a tree of your choice. Once the fever is tethered to the tree, you are to depart, never to return. Should you make the mistake of seeking out the tree again, the fever will break free of its bonds and leap back inside you.

A Flemish cure sends you to a willow tree early in the day, whereupon you are to tie three knots in one of its branches and say politely, "Good morning, old one, I give thee the cold; good morrow, old one." Then turn and walk away without looking back.

The use of the willow in the Flemish rite undoubtedly evolved from the fact that the tree was long used against a variety of maladies, among them rheumatism and fever-inducing illnesses. You'll recall from chapter three that its salicin content has been proven of value in the treatment of rheumatism. In addition to being a painkiller, salicin has long been recognized as being able to reduce a fever.

Trees are not the only objects of value in the magic of transference. A number of animals—cats, dogs, and spiders in particular—will serve you quite as well:

Have a family member or friend pass a black cat across your chest. Or feed the cat the remainder of a soup that you have just downed.

Feed a dog a pound of beef that has been boiled in your urine.

Place a live spider in a box to be suspended from your neck. Or simply place the spider in a box and set it down somewhere in the house. Or imprison the thing in a box or a cloth and then bind the arrangement to your left arm. In each instance, the ague will depart as the spider wastes away and dies.

Some spider cures are neither magical in nature nor linked to transference. They do, however, share a characteristic with the above urine recipe for your dog. They are downright nauseating. Just two examples are needed to prove the point:

Catch a live spider and encase it in a bit of bread that is then rolled into a small ball. While fasting from all other foods, swallow the "pill."

Insert a spider or a ball made of its web in an apple. Then eat the apple.

As repugnant as these treatments are, generations of people who have tended to themselves have sworn by them. One point must be made about the spider's web. Research in 1882 established that its centuries-old employment against not only ague but also asthma and a variety of other fever-inducing illnesses was of genuine value. Laboratory research that year unearthed the fact that the web contains a substance—arachnidin—that is a highly effective febrifuge.

Now, back to the magical cures. Like the above two spider remedies, many cures in your folk medicine chest have nothing to do with transference. In England and the United States, for instance, you might come upon the one that echoes the age-old faith in the powers of an object that has been responsible for so much death: wear a few chips from a gallows about the neck or somewhere next to the skin.

The chips serve a double purpose. They can not only cure the ague but render you immune to future attacks as well. To gain immunity, you can also observe the old European and United States custom of eating three hard-boiled eggs on Good Friday. If you're caught in a hailstorm, you can achieve the same end by scooping up and swallowing its first three stones.

BITES

I pray thee, let me and my fellow have a haire of the dog that bit us last night.

John Heywood (1497?–?1580)
Proverbs

The British writer Heywood was here addressing a barkeep and requesting a time-honored remedy for a hangover—a small drink of whatever it was that had intoxicated him and a friend the night before. The remedy itself is an imbiber's variation of an ancient cure for animal bites:

To heal a dogbite, pluck a hair from the offending dog, burn it, and place it on the wound. Or eat the hair after hiding it in a bread-and-butter sandwich.

You can also heal a dogbite by killing the animal, removing and boiling its liver, and then applying the liver to the injury.

A snakebite can be healed if you will simmer the fat of the reptile and cover the wound with it. Actually, the cure will work with the fat of any snake.

At work in these remedies is a system of healing based on what is called sympathetic magic. The system is grounded in the ancient—probably even prehistoric—idea that a sympathetic connection exists between the injured one and the creature or, as we'll see later, the object that caused the injury. Consequently, you can aid your recovery through a procedure that deals with both the injury and the injurious one.

Very likely because it is difficult—and often impossible in cases of insect nips and stings—to snare the creature responsible for the harm, sympathetic magic as it applies to bites is usually restricted to those by dogs and snakes. The majority of folk remedies for other bites call for treatments customarily aimed at drawing the poison out of the body. Here is a sampling of such cures, beginning with one that can be tried if you're unable—or unwilling—to corral the dog that attacked you:

> Simply place a slice of onion on the injury. The remedy dates back to the writings of Pliny the Elder. The onion also is said to be of value in the treatment of mosquito and other bites. At least, some English country people have long thought so.

As for snakebite, the American Indians have come up with a variety of plant cures. For example:

> Boil the leaves of the Carolina poplar and hold the wounded area over the rising steam.

> Cut open the fang marks so that the poison will escape in the flow of blood. You may also want to suck

the blood away. Then tie wet plantain leaves about the bitten area.

Chew the roots of either the Virginia snakeroot or the Seneca snakeroot plant to make a poultice for the wound.

The plantain remedy was an Indian favorite not only for snakebites but for those of spiders and other poisonous insects as well. When the early settlers learned of the Virginia snakeroot's powers as an antidote for snakebite, it became a highly popular European treatment for the bites of mad dogs. The Seneca snakeroot was given the botanical name *Polygala Senegra* in honor of the Seneca tribe (*Senegra* is the Latin word for Seneca) who not only applied to it to snakebites but also brewed it in a tea to ease asthma and heart problems. The Virginia and Seneca varieties are not alone in being dubbed "snake" plants. White snakeroot was employed for centuries in Europe against poisons and venomous bites, with its botanical name, *Eupatorium rugosum*, referring to Mithradates Eupator (132–63 B.C.; sometimes spelled *Mithridates*), the king of the Black Sea realm, Pontus, who is said to have been the first man to have employed it as an antidote. The Algonquian Indians fashioned poultices of the crushed roots of the black snakeroot. The Navaho turned to the joe-pye plant, a relative of the white snakeroot, for snakebite and the wounds inflicted by poison arrows. The plant's name, however, has nothing to do with snakebite; rather the joe-pye is named for the Indian medicine man who made it famous in New England as a cure for typhus. Despite their use over the centuries, there is a problem concerning these plants. Their effectiveness as antidotes has never been proved conclusively.

And now what of other bites? What can be done about them? Here are some answers:

All poisonous insects: To draw out the venom from any poisonous bite, including that of a snake, place a live frog on the wound; when the frog dies, the poison will be gone.

Bee and wasp stings: If the stinger is left in the skin, remove it at once. Then coat the sting with honey (perhaps there is some sympathetic magic at work here). Or cover the sting with mashed ragwood, mud, or a quid of tobacco to soothe the pain and assist the healing. The juice from crushed chrysanthemum leaves can often bring relief when gently massaged into the pained area. A compound of baking soda and vinegar placed on the sting is an old southern folk remedy.

CONSTIPATION AND DIARRHEA

I've not looked forward to writing about the first of these two topics because it brings me face-to-face with the memory of a childhood medicinal ogre—castor oil. I count myself among the countless European and American children who, ever since the late eighteenth century, have been made to force the horrid stuff down past their innocent palates at the first sign of an intractable bowel or, as a matter of fact, any other complaint that turned them pale, listless, or ornery.

The oil is derived from the beans of the castor oil plant. The plant, which can range to heights of thirty to forty feet, originated in Africa and, in time, came to be cultivated in warm regions throughout the world. The history of its beans is as long as the taste of their oil is foul. They have been found in clusters in Egyptian tombs that predate the birth of Christ by some two thousand years. They were apparently put there to assist the distinguished corpse in three ways during his stay in the hereafter: to soothe his aches and pains, aid his digestive system, and provide him with light. The Egyptians used the beans for their lamps, made unguents of them, and purged their systems with them monthly—in fact, usually three times a month.

Though the Egyptians had no fear of the bean as a laxative, the same cannot be said of the Greeks and Romans. They recognized that it is poisonous, so much so that a single one is capable of killing a child. And so, though the Greeks used the bean at times as a purgative, both cultures pretty well restricted it to external problems, employing it as a liniment.

The Greek and Roman caution persisted until the late 1700s, when the oil extracted from the bean became universally fashionable as a laxative. The toxic substance in the beans and in all parts of the castor oil plant is called ricin. But the oil is quite safe when extracted commercially because, when the beans are crushed at a temperature below 100°F., the ricin does not mix with the resultant oil but remains in the residue left behind. The oil ends up being non-toxic and rich in another substance, *ricinolein*. Ricinolein works as a laxative by irritating the intestines and causing them to be rid of their contents.

Well, that's just fine. But, benign though it may be, the oil has an out-and-out rotten taste. What can you, in your bygone day, do to disguise its taste so that you or your child will be able to swallow the stuff? My mother's pet trick was to mix the oil with orange juice. But the two, like oil and water, are incompatible. They want nothing to do with each other. And so the oil would settle at the bottom of the glass and lie there, waiting in malignant glee as I approached that final, God-awful swallow.

Your medicine chest may have two solutions to the taste problem. For one, mix an ounce of glycerine with two drops of oil of cinnamon and then add an ounce of castor oil. I have a friend who remembers this concoction as tasting like candy.

The other advises that you can change the taste of the oil to that of fresh oysters by drinking a glass of water in which nails have been allowed to rust.

I have no idea whether these two systems work, and I have no intention of putting them to the test. I have always loathed even the thought of castor oil. And I'm not too fond of oysters or rusty nails either.

Through the centuries, numerous plants have been brewed into laxatives. Included on their roster are aloe (probably used sparingly because it can cause severe intestinal cramps), basil, fenugreek, licorice, and garlic. For centuries, the fig has proved a trustworthy aid. Much favored by the early settlers in the American West was a tea made of the boiled bark of the cascara sagrada plant (meaning "sacred bark" in Spanish); they learned of the bark's efficacy from the local Indians, who set it against various ailments but chiefly liked it for ending constipation and upset stomachs.

The cascara bark is an effective purgative because it houses two types of the substance anthraquinone. The first increases the movement in the large intestine, while the second affects a nerve center there. A fluid extracted from the bark has been marketed commercially since the 1870s.

Now let's say that you suffer a visit by constipation's exact opposite, diarrhea. Many a folk-medicine chest contains what may seem a strange remedy. It entails eating a food so spicy that it promises trouble rather than help. You're to nibble on one of the pod-like fruits of the cayenne pepper plant or mix it in with your dinner. It is said to work well because it contains the substance capsaicin. Capsaicin is the ingredient that burns your mouth, reddens your cheeks, and makes your eyes water, but it is also the ingredient that makes life unbearable for the bacteria causing diarrhea.

A less daring strategy is based on an old Christian belief: eat bread that has been baked on a Good Friday. The bread is thought to be blessed and to contain curative powers because of the religious significance of the day on which it is prepared. It was long the custom of English priests and wives to set aside loaves for use against various sicknesses throughout the entire year. They held that Good Friday bread never went moldy.

CUTS

Should you wound yourself, however slightly, when there is a spider web nearby, the object with a reputation for curing ague will now provide you with a handy remedy for stanching the flow of blood. Gather the web, roll it into a ball, and place it on the wound. The treatment and the styptic properties in the web have been admired since antiquity. Pliny the Elder wrote that the web could be used for an injury as serious as a fractured skull and a nick as minor as that made with a razor while shaving.

Once the flow of blood is controlled, you can turn to the system that reputedly works with dogbites and snakebites—sympathetic magic. The magic, you'll recall, is based on the age-old notion that a sympathetic connection exists between the injured party and whatever creature or object is responsible for the pain. In the case of an object, the whole idea seems to have originated in the fancy that the blood on the object continues to share a feeling with the blood in your body. You can take advantage of this connection and hasten your recovery not with the cruelty that is shown, say, to the snake—which must be killed to obtain the fat needed for healing—but by tending as much to the wounding object as to the wound.

Should you, for instance, accidentally pierce your hand or foot with a rusty nail, you can best help yourself by first cleansing the nail of rust and then polishing it to a sparkling brightness. Thereafter, it must be kept safely away from further use or harm.

Oil has long been a mainstay in the care given the wounding object in Great Britain and America. To avoid the dangers of infection, the farmer who cuts himself on a hook, a scythe, a nail, or a piece of wood will quickly coat the thing with oil and rub it to a glistening shine, often repeating the task daily. He will do the same thing to a thorn once he has removed it from his skin. It is not unusual for him to care for the object before he takes care of himself. Though oil has also been long employed in other societies, the British—and, subsequently, American—faith in it may have started with philosopher Sir Francis Bacon (1561–1626), who wrote: "It is constantly Received and Avouched that the Anointing of the weapon that maketh the Wound will heal the Wound it selfe." He then suggested a series of ingredients for the "Anointing" oil, some of them magical in nature and, to put it mildly, startling: "Moss upon the skull of a dead man unburied, and the fats of a boar or a bear killed in the act of generation." The "moss" is obviously usnea, the rheumatism cure mentioned in chapter three.

But what if you are one of the few of your time who want no traffic with magic? You'll then depend on several plant medications. You may choose to treat your wound by holding it in the steam coming from a sassafras root being boiled in water. You may opt for poultices made from the root bark of the bayberry. You may, as the ancients did, apply a liquid concocted by mixing sage leaves with white wine. Or you may decide to cover the injury with the bruised leaves of the plant thought so efficacious that it was early given the name woundwort.

The sassafras root, which is known to contain antiseptic properties, is perhaps the most effective of the above lot. The other plants may or may not prove beneficial. While they contain astringent substances (tannin in sage, for example) that make them useful in easing sore throats, there is doubt that they are of actual value in treating wounds, with future research necessary to resolve the matter one way or the other.

EARACHES

What was perhaps the most popular earache treatment available in bygone days is shocking to health-conscious people of the late twentieth century:

Have someone blow tobacco smoke into the pained ear.

There is some doubt that the tactic actually works. All that anyone can say is that it might—and sometimes does—bring relief.

Another old-time favorite advises that you:

Build a mound of black pepper on a tiny piece of cotton batting. Roll the batting into a wad, with the pepper locked inside, and dip it in castor, olive, or corn oil, after which it is to be placed in the ear opening. You'll then be wise to wrap a strip of flannel cloth about the head to keep the batting warm.

If, in your misery, this process seems a bit too complicated or time-consuming, you can simply pour the castor oil into the ear. At least you won't have to put up with its taste.

Warmth, as it does in the cotton-batting treatment, plays a role in several other cures. One example: roast an onion in wood coals and then insert its heart into the ear. Another: after roasting the onion, wet down the ear with drops of the warm juice.

If you have the nerve for it, try heating a spoonful of your urine and pouring a few drops into the ear. Or roast a strip of lean mutton, squeeze it dry, and let the resultant juice do the job. Or why not merely hold the pained ear close to a lighted lamp?

Finally, here's a cure with a dash of magic to it. Trap a weasel and have the oil from its ears ease the pain. Where's the magic? You'll be wasting your time unless the weasel is of your own sex.

EYE PROBLEMS

British country people have two distinctly opposite methods—one charming and the other disgusting—for tending troubled eyes. The first urges you to collect rain water that falls on Holy Thursday and place it in a clean bottle for future use. Like Good Friday bread, it is said to be blessed and a fine curative because of the day on which it falls.

The second, which can be traced back at least to the seventeenth century, is advised for blindness and any pain whatsoever in the eye:

> Begin with the head of a black cat, making certain that you can detect no other color in the fur. Burn the head to a powder. Then, three times a day, blow the powder into the sufferer's eyes by means of a straw or quill.

A not-quite-so-sickening—but nevertheless still sickening—variation of this treatment is used for curing the sty. Rub the sty with the tail of a dead cat.

What is undoubtedly the best-known cure for the sty is to massage it with a gold ring, preferably a wedding ring. The wedding ring is an obvious and practical folk choice because it is so readily at hand and entails no extra cost for the family. The use here of gold, which has been regarded worldwide as the most precious of metals since antiquity, is a leftover from its once-widespread employment in both folk and formal medicine. It was thought to be imbued with great healing properties because of its refusal to rust.

But there is also an ancient magic at work in the gold massage and another cure of almost equal fame—the pricking of the sty with a gooseberry thorn. In each instance, the sty is to be massaged or pricked either three or nine times. Both numbers enjoy an age-old mystical significance in societies across the world.

The Greek philosopher Pythagoras (c. 580–500 B.C.), made three the symbol of deity, calling it the perfect number because it is expressive of "beginning, middle, and end." In the Christian faith, it came to represent the Trinity; in a number of ancient societies it represented the ruling gods of the world—for the Romans, Jupiter (heaven), Neptune (the sea), and Pluto (the underworld); in India, the Brahmans gave their god three heads. The list goes on from there: the Greek and Roman Fates were three (controlling as they did birth, life, and death), as are the Christian Graces (Faith, Hope, and Charity); the world itself is threefold (land, sea, and sky); so is man (body, mind, and spirit); and so are his enemies (the world, the flesh, and the Devil). As for the number nine, among its mystical attributes it has the distinctions of being the trinity of trinities and the plural trinity.

It would be doing both numbers an injustice to mention them solely in connection with making the commonplace sty go away. They have long played a vital role in various cures. To name just one, an old European and American remedy for dysentery requires the patient to dig up the root of a bramble bush, cut it into nine pieces, and hold them in his left hand while he sings the *Miserere* three times. They are then to be mixed with mugwort and boiled in milk, with the milk to be sipped at the end of a day's fasting.

No matter its promised efficacy, the pricking of the sty with a gooseberry thorn may hold little appeal for you. If so, you can put your faith in an Irish cure: point the thorn at the sty nine times while chanting "Away, away, away!"

A final mention must be made of gold. If you wish to sharpen your eyesight, do what generations of seamen have done for the same reason: wear gold earrings.

NOSEBLEEDS

As far as I can find, the folk-medicine chest contains no plant remedies for nosebleeds, perhaps because these commonplace bothers come so abruptly and often pass so quickly that you haven't the time to collect the needed plant. Instead, you're advised to:

Roll up a piece of paper and press it under the upper lip.

Wring out a cloth that has been soaked in hot water and spread it on the back of the neck.

Lay a cold, damp cloth across the forehead and nose. For best results, make certain that your hands have first been soaked in cold water and that you apply a bottle of hot water to the patient's feet.

Aside from these approaches, most cures advise the use of metal objects and strings. First, the "metal" cures:

> As soon as the bleeding commences, place a pair of scissors flat against the back of the neck and press them against the skin. In some regions, the scissors are to be placed with their points turned upwards.

> If you prefer, press a nickel (in a variation of the rolled-paper technique) between the gum and the skin beneath the nose.

> Simpler yet: have the patient lie down. Then place a dime over his or her heart.

Most likely responsible for these remedies is the already-mentioned respect felt by the ancients for iron as a curative. You'll recall Pliny the Elder's opinion that iron, on being dipped into water when white-hot, gathered the mystifying strength to heal wounds and cure various ills, among them rheumatism.

And now the "string" cures: a vintage European and American ploy calls for some string to be tied about the little finger once the nose begins to bleed. But, should one nostril bleed, you're to try the following:

> If the left nostril is the one in trouble, tie the string about the little finger of the right hand. The string goes around the left little finger when the right nostril bleeds.

The ague-fighting spider is employed in an ugly British cure—now understandably out of fashion. The treatment was described by the sixteenth-century writer Thomas Lupton in his book, *A Thousand Notable Things, of Sundry Sortes*:

> If a Spider be put in a lynnen cloath a lytle brused, and holden to the nose that bleedes . . . by & by the bloud wil stay, and the nose wil leave bleeding . . . The venomous Spyder is so contrary, and such an enemie to man's bloud, that the bloud drawes back.

Folk medicine holds that nosebleeds, in common with virtually all other health complaints, can be prevented as well as cured. The traditional preventive is a charm suspended from a length of cord, string, or red woolen yarn and worn as a necklace. Your choice of an effective charm will depend much on where you live. If you're among the French in Louisiana, you'll opt for a key; in Europe and parts of the American South, pot hooks or a small chunk of lead with a hole bored through it; and in the Ozarks, glass beads or a nutmeg. Up in New England, the length of red woolen yarn by itself will do the trick. (Remember, as was said earlier, the color red symbolized magic for our forebears and was thought to be imbued with a mysterious strength to heal a variety of ills.)

TOOTHACHE

The folk treatments for toothache run the gamut from the practical—and often helpful—to the fanciful. One of the most practical of all has been a familiar in western folk and formal medicine since the fourth century A.D., when the dried leaves of the clove tree began arriving in Europe via the Arabian trade routes. Ever since, a simple home treatment has been to place the bruised leaves in the mouth. It's a remedy that works to some degree because the leaves are known to contain a mild antiseptic. At times, modern dentists mix oil of clove with zinc when making temporary fillings.

At least a dozen other plants and trees have been summoned through the centuries to ease the pain of a misbehaving tooth, among them calendula, mustard, plantain, oregano, and garlic. Oregano's employment can be traced back at least to Europe's medieval days. Should you turn to oregano, all you'll need do is massage the tooth and the adjoining gum area with the oil from its leaves. The relief, however, may be psychological rather than physical. There is no scientific evidence that the treatment actually works. On the other hand, there is no evidence that it doesn't.

Numerous societies have used garlic—and still do—for general health and to fight a host of ills. It once held an extra bonus for Europeans: it drove off vampires, ghosts, and evil spirits. But, so far as toothache is concerned, there is a problem similar to that posed by oregano. While research has shown that garlic contains antiseptic and antispasmodic properties that may make it an effective medicinal for a variety of ills (twentieth-century medicine is looking into its possible value in the treatment of cardiac and circulatory problems), there is nothing yet in modern research to justify the enduring faith it has earned as a toothache curative.

The American Indians put their trust in the prickly ash tree—so much so that they christened it the toothache tree. Their remedy was either to chew the bark or to crush it into a pulp that was then held against the pained area. As far as a nineteenth-century European naturalist was concerned, however, their confidence was misplaced. During his study of native American plants, he experimented with the bark on a tooth of his own and disgustedly wrote that it did no lasting good. It succeeded only in burning his mouth so badly that he forgot his pain for a while. Then, back came the ache.

At least in part, the reasoning behind the Indian use of the irritating prickly ash may have been the same as the reasoning that inspired the cures for a host of ills—the conviction that the worse-tasting or worse-appearing a medicine is, the better it will work. Galen (A.D. 129–200) of Greece, whose medical reputation ranks right alongside that of Hippocrates, prescribed boiling a frog in water and vinegar and then holding the little creature in the mouth. What will certainly strike many as the most loathsome of toothache medicines was a European staple for centuries: a mouthful of one's own urine.

The above two treatments were not chosen simply because they are repugnant. Both are fanciful and stem from the ancient notion that both the frog and the urine (human and animal alike) possessed magical powers—this despite the fact that the frog was widely thought to bestow warts on anyone who touched it (but, in itself, was that not a sign of some magic potency?). Just as fanciful—but quite understandable because it was based on the ancient awe of the power triggered by one of nature's most frightening spectacles—was a cure reported by Pliny the Elder in his *Natural History* and then employed right up to the twentieth century:

Find a tree that has been struck by lightning. Pull some of the bark away and press it against the tooth.

In Europe and America, a religious belief once played a major role in the treatment of tooth pain. It had to do with a legend that had sprung up about Jesus and St. Peter. According to the legend, as Jesus was passing through Jerusalem one day, he stopped to talk with an obviously unhappy and uncomfortable Peter. He asked the Apostle what was ailing him, to which Peter replied that he was suffering such a toothache that he could not stand, sit, lie, or walk. Jesus ended the pain by telling Peter to rise and follow him.

The legend (or variations of it) served for centuries—in fact, until well into the twentieth century—as a charm to end or avoid a toothache altogether. It required you to do no more than carry on your person a written account of the story or a prayer based on it.

A thirteenth-century variation of the legend had it that Mary, not Peter, was the sufferer, and that it was the Holy Ghost, not her son, who stopped to visit her. A later version named St. Thomas as the victim. Out of that version came the belief that a toothache could be put to flight by a healer who massaged the throbbing area with a rock while reciting the words that Christ spoke to Thomas at the time:

Thomas, swear now for My sake
And you shall never have toothache.

But what of the methods for preventing toothache in the first place? They are simplicity itself, with none having a thing to do with religious belief. One of the simplest comes from New England, and has always struck me as an infallible sign of Yankee ingenuity. All you need do is trim your fingernails on a Friday. You will then not be troubled by toothache throughout the coming week. Repeat the process each Friday for a lifetime free of tooth pain.

One of the tastiest ploys—at least, in the eyes of some people—likewise comes from New England. It only works, however, if you've just had your first tooth pulled. Place the extracted tooth in a glass of whiskey. Drink the whiskey. You'll never again be made to suffer a toothache that ends in the tooth being pulled.

Then there are these two European and American approaches:

When dressing, always remember to put your left stocking and shoe on first. Your care here will prevent not only toothache, but an array of other ills as well—not to mention plain old bad luck.

Go about with the gall of a rose in your clothing. The gall is a swelling of a plant's tissue and is usually caused by fungi or other parasites.

WHOOPING COUGH

Whooping cough is an infectious disease that, following an incubation period of two weeks or so, brings on fits of coughing that persist for another three weeks to a month. The paroxysms, which can trigger vomiting and hemorrhaging, are agonizing for the patient and a test of the patience of anyone who must listen to them day and night. The number of paroxysms can range from ten in a twenty-four hour period to between forty and fifty. A highly contagious disease, whooping cough most often strikes children.

Folk medications for relieving the paroxysms have been on the scene for centuries. When your child falls victim to whooping cough, some of the most venerable and admired of their number advise that you:

Heat turpentine and carbolic acid and have the youngster inhale their fumes.

After boiling chestnut leaves in water, drain away the water, flavor it with honey, and administer the concoction as a drink. Honey, with its soothing mucilage content, has been used for coughs of every description since antiquity.

Make a paste of garlic and lard and massage it into the patient's back and chest.

Brew the leaves of the thyme plant in water to make a tea for the child. This medication may be the best of the lot. Thyme contains both antispasmodic and antitussive properties.

Of course, magical cures were also available. Always at your disposal is transference. You can conjure up its wonders by trapping any of several small animals and, while they are still alive, having the patient wear them as necklaces or carry them somewhere in their clothing. For instance, a black beetle imprisoned in a folded cloth or small box is an old-time favorite. So is the ague-fighting spider when it is placed between two walnut shells. The same holds true for the caterpillar tied away in a small bag. In each instance, the coughing spells dwindle as the trapped creature wastes away to death.

A nasty transference trick can be pulled on a neighborhood dog. Cut several hairs from your child's head. Hide them in a wad of butter that you then give to the unsuspecting animal. Once the butter is swallowed, the dog will take the disease, your youngster will return to good health, and you'll be in for your first decent night's sleep in weeks.

The family cat can also be enlisted, but not for the purposes of transference. Pluck nine hairs (that magic number again) from the animal, cut them into pieces, and dip them in water to be drunk by the patient.

If you're able to trap a ferret, fetch a saucer of milk for the prisoner and allow him to lap up just a portion. The remainder goes to your young patient.

What has always struck me as one of the oddest of whooping-cough cures has long been in use in Great Britain. (The cure will still be trusted by some country people in the twentieth century.) It advises you to keep an eye out for a man riding a piebald horse. On glimpsing his steed, you're to hurry to him and ask how the disease can be cured. For some mysterious reason, he is supposed to know the correct answer.

I have no knowledge of why the rider is expected to provide an infallible remedy. My guess is that the whole fancy may have started with the coincidence of a worried parent asking after a cure from a friend who happened to be mounted on a piebald horse at the time. The rider suggested a medication or ritual that may have actually brought relief or seemed to work because the patient was about to recover anyway. From that moment on, the word of the rider's uncanny ability spread throughout the surrounding regions. As was said in earlier passages, many folk remedies undoubtedly took shape and then fanned out not just to the nearby hills and valleys but to the entire world as a result of the "magic" of coincidence.

For two chapters now, we've talked as if you lived in a bygone age. Now we return to our own time for a look back at the ideas and ideals that guided our forebears in answering a question that has been asked since antiquity and that is second to none in importance in folk medicine. It was a question as vital to past generations as it is to us in our health-conscious late twentieth century with all its medical wonders, all its research, and all its sometimes-tiring emphasis on proper diet, prudent living habits, and sufficient physical exercise:

How can one live a long and healthy life?

Some Thoughts on Illness

Prevention is better than cure.

> Desiderius Erasmus (1466–1536)

The modern variation:

An ounce of prevention is worth a pound of cure.

A disease known is a disease half cured.

> Europe and America

Some remedies are worse than the disease.

> Publilius Syrus (1st century B.C.)

Desperate diseases require desperate measures.

> England and the United States

There is one topic peremptorily forbidden to all well-bred, to all rational mortals, namely, their distempers. If you have not slept, or if you have slept, or if you have headache, sciatica, or leprosy, or thunderstroke, I beseech you, by all angels, to hold your peace.

> *The Conduct of Life*
> Ralph Waldo Emerson (1803–1882)

Patience is the cure for all illness.

A long disease doesn't tell a lie;
It kills at last.

Irish proverb

A hypochondriac: One who's afraid he's sick and dead scared that he's not.

And this variation of the old saying about cowards and heroes:

The ordinary man dies but once;
A hypochondriac a thousand imes.

Still another variation, this one a play on the saying about the religious zealot being one who is afraid that somewhere, somehow, and at some time, someone is having a good time:

A hypochondriac is one who is terribly afraid that somewhere, somehow, and at some time in his body, something is working as it should.

Now to close with a gentle truth:

The sickness of the body
May prove the health of the soul.

CHAPTER SEVEN

To Your Health

CERTAINLY AS MUCH AS, and perhaps even more than, we in this health-conscious late twentieth century, our fore-bears—without today's medical marvels, without today's medical insurance, faced with an alarmingly brief life-span, and with physicians who too often worked in a sci-entific half-light and in the darkness of superstition—recognized not only the dangers of illness but also, of even greater importance, the benefits of a robust health. This recognition is more than evident in the axioms and com-ments that have have come down to us from virtually every era and society. A smattering of examples:

He who has health has hope,
And he who has hope has all.

Arabian proverb

Good health and good sense are two of life's greatest blessings.

Rome
Publilius Syrus (1st Century B.C.)

The first wealth is health.

United States
The Conduct of Life
Ralph Waldo Emerson (1803–1882)

151

* * *

O health, health! the blessing of the rich! the riches
of the poor! who can buy thee at too dear a rate, since
there is no enjoying this world without thee?

> England
> *Volpone*
> Ben Jonson (1572–1637)

His best companions, innocence and health:
And his best riches, ignorance of wealth.

> England
> *The Deserted Village*
> Oliver Goldsmith (1730–1774)

Health is better than wealth.

> Irish proverb

Ill-health, of body or of mind, is defeat. . . .
Health alone is victory.

> England
> Thomas Carlyle (1795–1881)

Throughout this book, we've talked of the methods
our forebears employed to prevent as well as cure specific ailments and diseases. In this chapter, we turn to
what they had to say to anyone who wished to live a
healthy and, as a consequence, long life. The suggestions range from general admonitions on remaining
healthy and avoiding illness to comments on our eating,
drinking, smoking, and sleeping habits. The observa-
tions come from the most common of folk at one end
of the scale to some of the most distinguished figures
in history at the other.

ON LEADING A HEALTHY LIFE

For Americans, there is probably no general counsel for insuring our physical health—plus, for good measure, our financial and intellectual well-being—more familiar than the everyday wisdom that made its debut in a 1758 edition of *Poor Richard's Almanac*:

> Early to bed and early to rise
> Makes a man healthy, wealthy, and wise.
> > Benjamin Franklin (1706–1790)

The phrase "early to rise" suggests that Franklin also believed in the idea of work as a guarantor of good health. If so, he would have seen eye-to-eye with a fellow American of a later age, social reformer Wendell Phillips (1811–1884), who commented:

> Health lies in labor, and there is no royal road to it but through toil.

Proponents of the Christian ethic and its emphasis on hard work have never had trouble with the Phillips view. The same can be said of any believer in the values of positive thinking who comes upon the following blunt advice by English author and statesman Edward Bulwer-Lytton, 1st Earl of Lytton (1831–1891):

> Refuse to be ill. Never tell people you are ill; never own it to yourself. Illness is one of those things which a man should resist on principle at the outset.

According to England's Sir Francis Bacon (1561–1626), good health is not only to be found in a positive outlook, but also in thinking for ourselves. He advised that we not depend on the likes, dislikes, and fears of others to guide us in living our lives. Rather, we should decide for ourselves what serves us best:

> There is wisdom in this beyond the rules of physic. A man's own observation, what he finds good of and what he finds hurt of, is the best physic to preserve health.
>
> *Of Regimen of Health*

Much of the folk advice for maintaining health is quite specific and calls for prudence on the part of the healthy when visiting or attending the ill. Here are three of the best known and still observed specifics:

Do not come near a contagious disease on an empty stomach.

Do not sit between a sick person and a fire. The heat will attract the vapors to you.

Do not enter a sickroom when you are warm and perspiring. Your pores will attract the sickness as you cool.

Of the trio, the third has always struck me as being a common-sense wisdom. But folk medicine would not be folk medicine without its share of eccentricities. And so we have more specifics, again three:

Do not allow a youngster to sleep with Grandma, Grandpa, or any elderly person. The elderly sleeper will draw off the strength and vitality of the young one. In fact, it's a no-win situation all around. The child will weaken and the elderly person gain nothing from the transference.

Never allow a cat to creep into bed with anyone—neither adult nor child, especially a child. The creature will suck the human's breath away.

For a lifetime of good health, always sleep with your head either to the north or the east.

The fear that a cat is able to suck the breath out of a sleeper is traceable to the Europe of the Middle Ages, a hotbed of grim attitudes and grimmer superstitions if there ever was one. In antiquity, the cat was regarded as a sacred animal and was much revered. But not in early Christian Europe. There, it became associated with the likes of witches, ghosts, and evil spirits, with the result that it became the subject of numerous ugly superstitions. Not only could it suck the breath from a sleeping human, but it could also turn a corpse into a vampire, indicate a hard voyage for a ship's crew by constantly mewing, and, if it were black, bring bad luck simply by crossing one's path in Germany, England, and later the United States. For many people of the day, it was Satan, a witch, or the shade of a dead person in disguise.

In antiquity, the cat was viewed and revered as a sacred animal in great part because of its regal mien and its agility. Two still-surviving notions come from this regard. First, the superstitions that rheumatism will strike anyone who kicks a cat and that Satan will attack anyone who drowns the animal are undoubtedly echoes of the ancient belief that supernatural retribution invariably follows the defilement of a sacred creature or object. Second, the idea that the cat has nine lives (a fancy no longer voiced seriously but nevertheless familiar to us all) is based on the animal's agility, especially its uncanny ability to land on its feet at the end of a fall.

Now, a note on the direction in which your head should be placed during sleep. According to some believers, the north is your best bet because the north magnetic pole lies in that direction. Others prefer the east, saying that it is the direction in which the earth is spinning, and that you're safest traveling headfirst through space.

To conclude, we leave the eccentric and return to the very practical for a compilation of health hints by those two writers we've mentioned at intervals in the preceding chapters, Mrs. Gillette and Mr. Ziemann, who seem to have something to say about everything in their 1887 *The White House Cook Book*:

Don't sleep in a draught.
Don't go to bed with cold feet.
Don't stand over hot-air registers.
Don't eat what you do not need, just save it.
Don't try to get cool too quickly after exercising.
Don't sleep in a room without ventilation of some kind.
Don't stuff a cold lest you should be next obliged to starve a fever.
Don't sit in a chilly room without a fire.

Don't try to get along without flannel underclothing in winter.

FOOD AND EATING

Tell me what you eat and I will tell you what you are.
Physiologie du goût
Anthelme Brillat-Savarin (1755–1826)

Man is what he eats.

We moderns interpret these two sayings as pertaining to the nutrition or lack of it in our various foods—namely, that the foods we choose can, for good or evil, dictate our appearance, affect our energies and sense of well-being, influence our personalities, and perhaps even determine the length of our lives. But, had the sayings been on the scene in antiquity, they would have meant something quite different for many cultures. The people would have interpreted them to mean that certain animals were to be eaten so that their admired characteristics could be passed into the human to endow him or her with the traits needed for both health and survival. This idea is an example of transference in one of its earliest forms, and is to be found even today in various primitive societies.

The animals used for these purposes were numerous. Parents in many cultures, both advanced and primitive, wrapped their infants in lion, tiger, and bear skins to arm them with the strength and ferocity necessary to fight off future illnesses. Both warriors and common folk, again in both advanced and primitive societies, ingested the lion's heart or blood, the jaguar's tail, and the eagle's wings for strength and courage. The Indians in some South American regions thought that they became more agile—and thus better hunters and fighters—when they ate monkeys and birds. A number of peoples believed that the eating of the sharp-eyed eagle would bless them with fine vision.

The age of an animal often played a role in transference. In Greek mythology, the sorceress Medea restored to youth the aged Aeson by feeding him the juices of various herbs, plus the liver of a long-lived deer and the head of a crow that had survived for more than nine generations of humans (Aeson was the father of Jason, the legendary figure who went in search of the Golden Fleece). Sir James Frazer, in his *The Golden Bough*, writes that when the Zulus of South Africa were struck by a serious disease, their medicine men would have both the sick and the well eat the bones of an aged animal so that they would survive to live as long as the animal had.

But there was disagreement among some peoples as to whether the characteristics in a given animal were to be desired or shunned. The Indians of North America ate the deer to acquire its fleetness, but it was taboo for the tribesmen in Borneo. They wanted no part of any deer because they looked on the animal as being too easily frightened.

The deer in Borneo was far from being the world's only taboo food. For example, as Sir James Frazer explains, again in *The Golden Bough*, the warriors of Madagascar were not allowed to eat either the hedgehog or the knee of the ox. The former was banned because the hedgehog's despised habit of coiling into a ball when frightened promised to curse the warrior with a timid disposition. The knee of the ox was known to be weak and so was to be avoided, lest the warrior's knees themselves weaken and collapse beneath him in battle or while on the march.

Frazer also points out that a food could be taboo without ever being eaten. Continuing with Madagascar as an example, he writes that the warrior there took care never to eat an animal that had been killed with a spear, or any cock that met its death while fighting; to eat the first would promise the warrior's death by a spear, and to eat the second prophesied his own death in battle. Further, his family was to slaughter no animal while he was away at war, for he would then die in battle—and perhaps at the very same moment of the animal's death. Nor did he dare eat kidney, for fear of being fatally shot, this because, in his language, the words for "kidney" and "shot" are the same. In other tribes, the people refused to eat a hare or hen lest they be rendered as timid as the two.

As ugly and as paradoxical as it may seem to us, it was common practice in tribal societies to cannibalize certain human enemies for the purpose of transference, and to feel that they were paying them the highest of compliments in doing so. When writing of a tribe in southeastern Africa, Frazer tells of how an especially courageous and formidable enemy, after being killed in battle, would have various parts of his body—among them the liver for valor, the ears for intelligence, and the testicles for strength—cut away and burned to ashes, with the ashes then being mixed into a paste that was fed to young tribesmen at the time of their initiation into adulthood.

Magic, as you know, was at the root of all transference practices. However, magic played no part in some other food taboos. The best known of these taboos comes to us from the ancient Jews and forbids the eating of those animals that are cloven-footed but not cud chewing—namely, swine. This prohibition against pork, which remains in Orthodox Jewish law, is recognized today as being a sound one medically. The ancient Jews did not know *why* pork was, as they put it, an "unclean food," but they could certainly see at first hand the harm it could do. It was not until centuries later that science uncovered the microbial *trichinella* parasites that lie coiled in cysts in the muscles of pigs. The parasites give the name trichinosis to the illness that can come of eating underdone pork.

The ancient Jews were also responsible for another common-sense dietary law. Before it could be eaten, an animal had to be killed by an approved ritual, which included draining the creature's blood away. No animal which had died naturally could be eaten. That the Jews knew what they were doing here is obvious in the fact that flesh quickly putrefies and becomes inedible, especially in the warm climate in which the Jews lived at the time. Further, no intelligent human, regardless of his time and place, needs to be told more than once of the dangers inherent in eating the flesh of any creature that has died of an unknown cause.

Turning now to foods other than flesh, we come immediately to what is assuredly the western world's most famous dietary axiom, following it with a lesser-known variation:

An apple a day keeps the doctor away.

Eat an apple going to bed,
Make the doctor beg his bread.

The above sayings appear to be well based in fact. The apple, to list just a few of its values, is known to contain pectin, which serves as a non-irritating stimulant that assists bowel elimination. It is also known to house vitamins in abundance, among them C for sound bones and teeth, B for healthy nerves, and G (riboflavin) for digestion and growth. It is recognized as a blood purifier, and has long been advised for low blood pressure and hardening of the arteries.

Aside from the apple axioms, there are just a few sayings that point out the values of certain diets, with a well-known one—at least in societies where wheat is the basic grain staple—coming from the pen of British writer Jonathan Swift (1667–1745):

Bread is the staff of life.

The Tale of a Tub

One of the oldest of European and American folk wisdoms advises an unusual food that promises a dual benefit—both good health and a long life. It urges us to eat the leaves of the sage plant.

Through the centuries, this plant has been made to serve many medical purposes. Its history has seen it employed to heal wounds and snakebites, cure the ague, ease sore throats, restore the sight, and whiten the teeth. But its greatest fame rests on its age-old reputation for guaranteeing a long life to those who make it a part of their diet.

The first word in its botanical name, *salvia officinalis*, is derived from the Latin for ''salvation.'' Two old sayings attest to the plant's reputed life-sustaining abilities:

> Why should a person die when sage grows in his garden?

> He that would live for aye
> Must eat sage in May.

The first of the two axioms can be traced back to medieval Europe, to the physicians serving with the great medical school at Italy's University of Salerno. The second calls for the plant to be eaten annually just prior to blooming. Its powers that insure one's longevity were said to be at their most potent at that time.

The link between the intake of sage and an extended life may have evolved from the fact that the plant survives for a long time after being plucked, a fact that early made the plant a symbol of endurance. Because of this many people of another day in England and America not only ate sage for longevity but placed it on graves as well, signifying that the departed would not be forgotten by friends and loved ones.

Early on, sage also became associated with wisdom, obviously because wisdom itself has been historically linked with old age (that is, until our own era, with its extravagant obeisance to youth). It is not a coincidence that the term *sage* is our synonym for a wise man and our adjective for a wise judgment.

On the opposite side of the fence, there are several adages that warn of the dangers of certain foods, with possibly the best known being:

Oysters are in season only in the months containing the letter R.

The saying urges you to eat oysters only from September, through April, and to avoid them the rest of the year, especially in the warming months of May and June and the summer months of July and August. A marine biologist tells me that this is neither wise nor necessary advice, contending that oysters can be eaten in any season. The saying may have gotten its start when people noticed that oysters are watery in the summer and contain only small amounts of glycogen (a chief carbohydrate storage material in animals) at that time. I'm not one to argue with scientific know-how, but don't try to get me to go near one of the things in the summertime. The memory of an long-ago unhappy July experience remains fresh in my mind to this day.

Far outnumbering all the axioms pertaining to specific foods are those that comment on good eating habits and damn the age-old and all-too-human misuse of food. First, on wise eating habits, we have the words of two distinguished ancients of like minds:

Thou should eat to live;
Not live to eat.

Cicero (106–43 B.C.)

Other men live to eat,
While I eat to live.

Socrates (c. 469–399 B.C.)

In common with the above two statements, comments on the dangers of the misuse of food begin deep in antiquity and march forward through the centuries, capturing the attention of some very respected minds along the way:

If you are surprised at the number of our maladies, count the number of our cooks.

Seneca (4 B.C.–A.D. 65)

Now learn what and how great benefits a temperate diet will bring along with it. In the first place, you will enjoy good health.

Satires
Horace (65–8 B.C.)

To be short, and sparing, at meals, that I may be fitter for business.

Things Necessary to be
Continually Had in Remembrance
Matthew Hale (1609–1676)

Indigestion is that inward fate
Which makes all Styx through one small liver flow.

Don Juan
George Gordon, Lord Byron (1788–1824)

By suppers more have been killed than Galen ever cured.

Jacula Prudentum
George Herbert (1593–1633)

Galen (A.D. 129–200) was the Greek physician whose fame equaled that of Hippocrates, and whose writings drew together the best of classical medicine and influenced European science through the medieval period up to the Renaissance.

No matter how well-known and admired the above authors may be, their views are pithily matched by the commonplace wisdoms that folk medicine has given us:

Whatsoever was the father of disease,
Ill diet was the mother.

Gluttony kills more than the sword.

Many dishes make many diseases.

Or a variation that is sure to please a vegetarian, though it can be loosely interpreted to mean many foods:

Much meat,
Much malady.

ALCOHOL AND DRINKING

On coming to alcohol, we run into some sharply divided opinions concerning its advantages and disadvantages. For example, in the responses of imbibers to the warnings of temperance proponents, we have these opinions:

Drink no longer water, but use a little wine for thy stomach's sake.

1 Timothy

Wine is the most healthful and most hygienic of beverages.

> Louis Pasteur (1822–1895)

There are more old drunkards than old doctors.

Bacchus' blessings are a treasure,
Drinking is the soldier's pleasure,
Rich the treasure, sweet the pleasure,
Sweet is pleasure after pain.

> *Alexander's Feast*
> John Dryden (1631–1700)

But, as an opening salvo from the opposing camp, there is this cautionary inscription on an old English headstone:

My grandfather was buried here,
My cousin Jane, and two uncles dear;
My father perished with inflammation in the thighs
And my sister dropped down dead in the Minories;
But the reason why I'm here interred,
According to my thinking,
Is owing to my good living and hard drinking;
If therefore, good Christians,
You wish to live long,
Don't drink too much wine, brandy, or anything strong.

For those unwilling to heed an experienced voice from the grave, we have these supporting admonitions:

You take your health once too often to the whiskey shop till it gets broken.

Irish proverb

All excess is ill, but drunkenness is the worst sort. It spoils health, dismounts the mind, and unmans men. It reveals secrets, is quarrelsome, lascivious, impudent, dangerous, and bad.

William Penn (1644–1718)

He who is master of his thirst is master of his health.

The habit of using ardent spirits by men in office has occasioned more injury to the public, and more trouble to me, than all other causes. Were I to commence my administration again, the first question I would ask respecting a candidate for office would be, Does he use ardent spirits?

Thomas Jefferson (1743–1826)

TOBACCO AND SMOKING

Tobacco, that notorious member (by today's standards) of the nightshade family and a native of the Americas, had recorded a centuries-old history before it was brought from the New World to the Old in the mid-sixteenth century. During his voyages into the Caribbean, Christopher Columbus noted the Indians' use of the plant's leaf for smoking. Some years later, in 1556, Frenchman Jean Nicot, who was serving as his nation's ambassador to Portugal, sent the seeds of the plant to his queen, Catherine de Medici, and won the distinction of having the genus of the tobacco family (a collection of some sixty different species of shrubs and herbs) named in his honor, *Nicotiana*, and of giving the English language that now-hated word, "nicotine." England's Sir Walter Raleigh is mistakenly thought to have introduced the plant into Europe. Actually, what he did was acquaint his homeland with it in 1565, nine years after its appearance in France.

As for the term *tobacco* itself, it evolved from the Spanish *tabaco*, which, in its turn, came from the Carib Indian language: it was the Carib word for the pipe in which the plant's leaves were smoked.

Tobacco was cultivated or gathered wild by the Indians of both North and South America, though this cannot be said of all the tribes. There is doubt that it was used by the tribes in the far north of the Americas, and is known to have been a stranger to the Eskimos until the arrival of white explorers. For many of the Indians who did employ the plant, it was considered to be sacred in nature. They smoked it for ceremonial purposes (a classic example being the smoking of the peace pipe), offered it to their gods in religious rites, and smoked, chewed, or sniffed it for a variety of medical problems. They turned to it, for example, to ease tension and relieve respiratory ills.

Tobacco first became popular as a general medicinal in Europe, but was soon being smoked, chewed, and sniffed for pleasure. As a purveyor of pleasure, it wasted no time in earning a dual reputation—as a God-given gift to human pleasure and as a thoroughly detestable commodity. A record of this dual reputation has come down to us in a collection of now vintage comments. To begin, there are these paeans on its behalf:

Tobacco, divine, rare, superexcellent tobacco, which goes far beyond all panaceas, potable gold and philosopher stones, a sovereign remedy to all diseases.

The Anatomy of Melancholy
Robert Burton (1577–1640)

A cigarette is the perfect type of a perfect pleasure. It is exquisite, and it leaves one unsatisfied. What more can you want?

The Picture of Dorian Gray
Oscar Wilde (1854–1900)

Sublime tobacco! which from east to west
Cheers the tar's labor or the Turkman's rest.

The Island
George Gordon, Lord Byron (1788–1824)

A lone man's companion, a bachelor's friend, a hungry man's food, a sad man's cordial, a wakeful man's sleep, and a chilly man's fire.

Westward Ho
Charles Kingsley (1819–1875)

If interpreted in a certain way, the words of one noted British author suggest that he differed little from today's smoker. They leave no doubt as to his love of tobacco, but do they not also perhaps hint that he perceived the health dangers we moderns see in smoking? I cannot say, but merely guess.

For thy sake, Tobacco, I
Would do anything but die.

A Farewell to Tobacco
Charles Lamb (1775–1834)

Spoken like a dedicated smoker about to quit. Now, some words that will gladden the hearts of the most zealous of anti-smoking advocates:

> Pernicious weed! whose scent fair annoys,
> Unfriendly to society's chief joys,
> The worst effect is banishing for hours
> The sex whose presence civilizes ours.

Conversation
William Cowper (1731–1800)

Three bad habits: drinking the glass, smoking the pipe, and scattering the dew late at night.

Irish proverb

The harshest anti-smoking comment I've been able to find was written by England's James I (1566–1625):

A custom loathsome to the eye, hateful to the nose, harmful to the brain, dangerous to the lungs, and in the black stinking fumes thereof nearest resembling the horrible Stygian smoke of the pit that is bottomless.

A Counterblast to Tobacco

As annoyed as he was, the British monarch's dudgeon was restricted to the written word. But other dignitaries of the day expressed their outrage with stronger measures. Howard W. Haggard, in his *Devils, Drugs, and Doctors*, writes that in 1624, the pope threatened to excommunicate any of the faithful who used snuff. A tougher stance was taken by the emperor of Russia: he ordered all users—or, as he called them, "tobacco drinkers"—to suffer slit noses, a whipping, and exile to Siberia. The Turkish government arrested smokers and condemned them to death.

ON SLEEP—ENOUGH AND TOO MUCH

Again, as in the matters of food and drink, we run into some sharply opposed opinions when we deal with the matter of sleep. Those people who trust in its healing properties, both physical and emotional, seem to outnumber those who either dislike or distrust it.

Sleep is the best medicine.

A good laugh and a long sleep,
The best cures in the doctor's book.

Irish proverb

He that can take rest is greater than he that can take cities.

Poor Richard's Almanac
Benjamin Franklin (1706–1790)

Sleep is a priceless treasure:
The more one has of it, the better it is.

Chinese proverb

O magic sleep! O comfortable bird,
That broodest o'er the troubled sea of the mind
Till it is hush'd and smooth.

Endymion
John Keats (1795–1821)

* * *

Sleep, rest of nature, O sleep, most gentle of the divinities, peace of the soul, thou at whose presence care disappears, who soothest hearts wearied with daily employment, and makest them strong again for labors.

Metamorphoses
Ovid (43 B.C.–A.D. 17)

And two entries in closing from Miguel de Cervantes (1547–1616):

Blessing on him that first invented sleep!

Don Quixote

Sleep is the best cure for waking troubles.

But now some words from those who do not look on sleep in such a happy fashion, especially if pursued and enjoyed to excess. They bluntly regard it as the thief of precious time.

He who sleeps all the morning,
May go begging in the afternoon.

Five hours sleeps the traveler,
Seven a scholar,
Eight a merchant,
And eleven a knave.

There will be enough sleeping in the grave.

Three misfortunes for man: a long morning sleep,

long visits by his neighbors, and bad fences.

Irish proverb

After all the pros and cons of our eating, drinking, and sleeping habits, what can be suggested as general rules for handling them—and, for that matter, all our earthly preoccupations—properly? Two answers come to mind. They just may say everything that needs to be said.

Man does not live by bread alone.

Matthew

Temperance is the best physic.

COLLECTIBLES

On the Human Body

A great nose indicates a great man—
Genial, courteous, intellectual,
Virile, courageous.

Cyrano de Bergerac
Edmond Rostand (1868–1918)

Nose, nose, nose, nose!
And who gave thee that jolly red nose?
Sinament and Ginger, Nutmegs and Cloves,
And that gave me my jolly red nose.

Deuteromelia
Thomas Ravenscroft (1583–1633)

Men and women whose hair forms a widow's peak
will outlive their spouses.

English superstition

A gray eye is a sly eye,
And roguish is a brown one;
Turn full upon me thy eye,—
Ah, how its wavelets drown one.
A blue eye is a true eye;
Mysterious is a dark one,
Which flashes like a spark-sun!
A black eye is the best one.

Oriental Poetry
William R. Alger (1822–1905)

* * *

Bags under the eyes are often a sign of dissipation.

European and American belief

Dark circles under the eyes are often a sign of poor health, tiredness, or dissipation.

A universal belief

He has cut his eyeteeth: Referring to someone who is experienced and worldly-wise, this old saying stems from the fact that the eyeteeth are cut late, with the first set appearing at around sixteen months of age, and the second at about twelve years.

Wisdom Teeth: As with the above saying, the name given these teeth is based on the idea that wisdom is associated with maturity. Bearing the popular name for the third molars, the wisdom teeth appear late in life, usually somewhere between ages seventeen and twenty-five. Consequently, by the time of their arrival, the owner (though you might never know it in some cases) is expected to have acquired some degree of wisdom.

Cut your fingernails on:
Monday for health,
Tuesday for wealth,
Wednesday for news,
Thursday for shoes,
Friday for sorrow,
Saturday, a true love tomorrow.

The above is just one version of this long-familiar folk rhyme. Another has it that paring the nails on:

Monday brings news,
Tuesday brings new shoes,
Wednesday makes you travel,
Thursday brings more shoes,
Friday brings money,
Saturday brings your lover on Sunday.

Still other versions hold that trimming the nails on Thursday will bring illness, while a Friday trim will fetch a toothache. Sunday trimming promises the greatest travails, perhaps because of the old Christian ban on work of any sort that day. You'll end up in a fight or see blood before the next morning. Worse, you'll be fated to have Satan catch you at some future time.

A cheerful face is nearly as good for the invalid as healthy weather.

                              Benjamin Franklin (1706–1790)

There's no art
To find the mind's construction in the face.

                                        Macbeth
                              William Shakespeare (1564–1616)

Keep your mouth shut,
And your eyes, ears, and bowels open.

                                        old army saying

CHAPTER EIGHT

The Folk Doctor

UP TO THIS POINT, as promised in the introduction, we've talked mainly of folk medicine as it has long been practiced by families who have tended to themselves in the absence of formal medical care or in the reluctance—for reasons extending from financial hardship to distrust—to take advantage of that care. But this is not to say that folk medicine has been without its own doctors. As has been the case for eons, they are found throughout the world today. Working chiefly in primitive and tribal cultures and in certain ethnic and religious groups, they provide care that ranges from treating individual illnesses to battling community and regional epidemics. They are known to us by the general and, as we'll see, inadequate term, *medicine men*. It is to them and their work that we now turn.

AT THE DAWN: MEDICINE AND DOCTORS

Diseases, malfunctions of the body, and injuries have been the lot of living beings since the dawn of time. Because the world went without the written word for millions of years, there is no record at hand to substantiate this statement. But there is much other evidence to attest to its truth. Consider:

Late in the nineteenth century, in the windswept

regions of Wyoming, American paleontologist Roy Moodie unearthed a small chunk of bone from the tail of a dinosaur; the bone, once housed in an animal that lived in the Mesozoic period, bore the twisted outcropping of a tumor. Other fossils from prehistoric times have been scarred with the markings and distortions of such still-familiar maladies as arthritis and what may have been osteomyelitis. Egyptian mummies from recorded history, on being examined, have revealed the telltale signs of surgeries, rheumatism, and tuberculosis of the spine.

Certainly at the very dawn of time both animals and humans, throbbing with the instinctual desire to survive, learned to care for themselves, with the animals learning to seek out cold water when feverish, to lick their wounds, and to understand that certain plants can compensate for deficiencies in their diets. Humans learned to tend their wounds and found, through trial and error, which foods could poison, which could help to cure, and which could sustain health. But humans took a step that the animal could not take. Blessed with an intellect that extended far beyond instinct, they began to wonder *why* they fell ill.

From studies that have been made of primitive peoples who live and believe today much as their ancestors did eons ago, we know that the human mind attempted to answer that *why* deep in prehistory and came up with one of the world's first major concepts on the cause of illness. The concept, you'll recall from the introduction, held that disease resulted from two circumstances. Either something bad got into the body, or something good was taken out of it. As first conceived, the agents that got inside the body were frightening creatures—

demons, devils, evil spirits, imps, and the like. They were often sent to do their terrible work by a god seeking revenge on a human who had angered him with an insult, a snub, or some other inappropriate behavior. Just as often, they acted on their own; let a man walk where they lurked (and they lurked everywhere in antiquity) and he could count on one or more of their number leaping into his body to sicken him by staying for a time or by stealing away his strength, vitality, or his soul. Also widely held was the belief that the soul could thoughtlessly wander off or run away for some reason, in either case escaping the patient via an opening in the body, perhaps the pores, but usually the mouth, nose, or ears.

As time wore on, the number of causal agents grew and took many different forms. In the Americas, for instance, the Papago Indians of Mexico and the southwestern United States developed the idea that the spirits of the dead caused nervous disorders. The Iroquois believed that the spirit Buffalo brought rheumatism. The Seminoles and the Indians of the Carolinas steadfastly refused to kill a snake, for fear that its soul would prompt its relatives to attack and sicken or kill the murderer's loved ones. For the same reason, the Cherokees would not kill a wolf. And they would never spit into a fire, certain that its god would be insulted and visit them with toothache.

The violation of a society's customs, manners, and rituals also became a sure way for one to fall ill and die. In many parts of Africa today, it is still taboo to touch anything connected with the meals served to the tribal chief or king. His plate, utensils, and food are all sacrosanct. Whoever touches them, either knowingly or innocently, is doomed, with death due to come within a few days or weeks. The power of suggestion is so strong among those raised with this prohibition that many who have violated it have wasted away and died for no apparent physical reason.

The eating of foods other than those intended for royalty likewise could trigger illness. Often, the forbidden food was that of an animal regarded as sacred. Deep in the Pacific, the Tahitians worshipped the hermit crab, contending that anyone who ate the creature risked death. In cases of all food violations, however, most peoples contrived methods for sidestepping the death sentence. Chants, prayers, and purification rituals usually did the trick. A Tahitian could safely eat the hermit crab if he performed certain prescribed rites prior to getting down to his meal.

Early on, human enemies joined the list of health hazards, and were also to be feared as the bringers of illness. Certain primitive peoples living today as their ancestors did in Australia, Indonesia, and New Guinea fear a rope dangling from a tree; they say that an enemy put it there to snatch their souls away. In the Middle Ages and for centuries thereafter, countless Europeans believed that some of their neighbors—witches—could conjure up not only ill fortune but also madness, sickness, injury, and death. But, the human mind being the contradictory thing it is, these fearsome creatures were also thought able to do good. They were said to have a knowledge of drugs and could use them to heal (if they wished) and devise love and fertility potions.

Soon after man developed his first idea on the cause of illness (an idea that is widely viewed today as superstitious hokum but was really an intellectual and imaginative triumph, coming as it did at a time when the human mind was yet an infant and the world a darkly mysterious place), he gave birth to the practice of medicine. For some clue as to how long ago that practice took shape, we turn to *Les Trois Freres*, the Cave of the Three Brothers, in France. High on its walls looms the painted figure of a strange man-like creature. The figure is the work of a forever-anonymous Cro-Magnon artist sometime around 20,000 years ago.

The creature is imposing, even frightening. His head is decorated with the antlers of a stag. Wrapped about his body is an animal skin, possibly that of a bison or bear. He has the tail of a horse, the paws of a bear, and the ears of what is perhaps a wolf. His arms and legs are painted with stripes. His feet are those of a human. He seems to be dancing, his body thrust forward, his feet lifted, and his arms extended. His eyes, almost perfectly round, stare out unblinkingly at the viewer.

Scholars believe that the creature is not a nightmarish figment of the artist's imagination but the representation of an actual man, the physician of the day dressed in the robes of his profession (the word "profession" is not ill-advised here; physicians are widely regarded as the world's first professional class). The scholars call him the Sorcerer and look on him as the Adam of all doctors—a breed that advances onward from him through the ages to today's representatives in their smocks, surgical gowns, and masks.

Along the way, however, the world's physicians became separated into two branches, one being manned by those whose practices can be directly linked to the evolution of formal medicine. Their ranks have included such figures as the priest-physicians of Egypt,

Hippocrates of Greece, Galen of Rome (though he was a Greek), Ambroise Paré of France, John Hunter and Joseph Lister of Great Britain, and Benjamin Rush and Elizabeth Blackwell of the United States; and their history has been one of a sometimes steady, sometimes erratic, sometimes brilliant, and sometimes benighted advance from the darkness of scientific understanding to the light. The other was made up of those who practiced, as they still do today, folk medicine in its various forms and are known worldwide by that general term, medicine men.

THE MEDICINE MAN

As a general term, medicine men—or, as we'll use it from now on, medicine man—suffers from inadequacy on two counts when we must speak in specifics. First, it was initially used during the early exploration of the New World to describe any American Indian who treated the sick, performed such wonders as predicting or influencing the course of future events, or was blessed with characteristics that suggested magical or supernatural powers. From there, it was expanded in popular literature to include all folk practitioners, but subsequent research into the world's primitive and tribal societies has shown that the folk doctor, depending on where he practiced and often on how he practiced, was known to his people by a variety of names. In some societies, he might indeed be called the medicine man. In others, he bore, and still bears, a variety of names. Here is a representative list of his titles, along with the people he serves.

Shaman: Seen throughout Europe centuries ago, the shaman is now found chiefly in Siberia, Asia, the Arctic, the South Pacific, and regions of the Americas.

Curandero: He is the folk doctor to the Hispanic people of the southwest United States, Mexico, and Central America.

Man of Mystery: The name by which the medicine man was known to the Omaha Indians of North America.

Angalok: The doctor to the Eskimos.

Voodoo Doctor: The name given to the doctor who practices among the believers in the religion voodooism, chiefly among blacks in Africa, Haiti, and the southern United States.

Sorcerer: The medicine man as he is known in various regions, among them the South Pacific.

Second, the term is a misnomer because the ranks of the medicine man have included both men and women. Both sexes function as shamans, though they are usually not found together in a given society. There are *curanderos* and *curanderas*, and male and female voodoo doctors. Even in the ranks of midwives, those health providers who are neither folk nor professional doctors, there are men as well as women.

(I must insert two brief notes at this point. First, though both sexes are involved, I'm going to refer to the various folk practitioners as males, not out of a masculine arrogance but for ease of explanation. Second, I'm going to speak mostly in the past tense when describing the medicine man's work, this to avoid muddying the text with constant reminders that such-and-such a cure was attempted in the past and that another is still attempted today. Please remember, however, that many of the medicine man's practices, especially those of the shaman and the North American Indian doctor who deals in plant cures, are still in use today.)

Early on, the medicine man divided his work into three general steps. To begin, he had to win his patient's trust; even at the dawn of time, this was understood to be vital to the patient's recovery. Next, of course, he had to deal with the illness itself, first diagnosing the problem and then treating it. Finally, in the wake of a cure, he usually left behind some token that was intended to remind the patient of the miracle that had been wrought and to assure him that he was now safe from a similar attack in the future. The token might be an amulet or the instruction to abstain from a certain food or avoid certain places where the demon of a given illness was thought to lurk. In this third step and, as we'll see, in his methods of building patient trust and effecting a cure, the medicine man was every inch as much a doctor of the mind—in his own way, a psychologist or psychiatrist—as he was a doctor of the body.

Building Patient Trust

The reputation of an accomplished medicine man preceded him and laid the groundwork for his patient's trust before he arrived at the sickbed. But many of his colleagues, though not all, did not let matters rest there.

In common with their earliest forerunner, the Sorcerer, they adopted a professional dress, often settling on an outfit that was a variation of his: animal skins cloaking the body and decorating the head, perhaps the mask of an animal covering the face, perhaps paws or claws encasing the hands. All this finery, they knew, added immeasureably to the patient confidence so necessary for successful treatment.

They knew this because they understood how deeply their people, living as close to nature as they did, respected the animal life around them and feared many of its breeds, especially the ferocious and the poisonous. The respect was seen in the fact that people everywhere in antiquity—in both primitive and advanced societies—revered many, if not virtually all, of the animals around them as sacred creatures endowed with magical powers because of talents and capabilities far beyond those of the human: some were stronger than mere man, some could run faster, some could endure the cold better, some could fly, some could survive beneath the ground or in the water. All the deeply-held respect and fright could not help but be transformed into confidence in the medicine man's powers when the patient saw him looming above the sickbed and ready to fight whatever force was reponsible for the illness with the animal's sacredness, magical prowess, physical strength, and ferocity.

The faith in animals extended beyond the garb of many medicine men and served as a basis for their practice. Various native and tribal societies have long believed that certain animals themselves, as sacred creatures, have the ability to render cures. Prominent among these curers have been the bear, the badger, the rattlesnake, and the eagle. In the eyes of a number of United States Indian tribes—for one, the Zuni of our Southwest—the spirit Bear is considered the most powerful of all curers and is able to determine the illness at hand and the required course of treatment. Another spirit animal, Badger, is likewise revered by the Zuni, Hopi, and other tribes. It is especially trusted by the tribal women when birthing. They either wear or keep close by a badger paw in the hope that the animal's talent for digging its way out of the ground will assist them.

Diagnosis and Treatment

For the medicine man, the diagnosis and treatment of an illness have always depended much on magic and have assumed a variety of forms through the centuries. One of the oldest of his diagnostic techniques was *hepatoscopy*, the attempt to divine future events—among them the course an illness was due to run—through a study of the liver of an animal, often a goat, a chicken, or a sheep. The procedure, whose name comes from the Greek for liver, *hepar*, was known to the Babylonians some three thousand years before Christ, and then to the Greeks, Etruscans, and Romans; also familiar with it early on were peoples in Southeast Asia, Africa, and Borneo.

Hepatoscopy called for the animal to be sacrificed by the patient's family, after which its carcass was opened and the liver examined to see what it prophesied. The liver was used because, gorged with blood as it is, it was thought to be the seat of the soul and the source of vitality. If, on examination, the organ proved to be malformed in any way, a long illness lay ahead for the patient. If a blood vessel ran in one direction, recovery was promised, but death if it traveled in another direction. Should the liver be marked with a tumor, death was a certainty.

Diagnosis could also be accomplished by other magical means. In ancient China, oracle bones were consulted; these were animal bones on which questions concerning the patient were inscribed and then held over a fire until they cracked, with the various patterns etched by the cracks providing the answers to the questions. Elsewhere, the medicine man might, in any combination, perform dances, sing chants, or beat a drum to summon a spirit that would point out the nature of the illness and then assist in its cure. In those societies that revered the spirit Bear, the medicine man slipped his hand into a bear-paw glove and magically became the spirit itself, possessed of all its healing talents. The shaman would begin his work (as he still does) by entering into a trance and traveling to the spirit world, there to consult with "spirit helpers" who advised him on what to do with his patient. It is this alleged ability to enter the spirit world itself and not simply summon help from that world that principally distinguishes the shaman from most of his fellow practitioners.

Once the nature of the illness had been determined—and for the moment let us say that invading demons are at fault—the medicine man, by himself or with the aid of a spirit being, could then marshal a host of treatments, all of them magical, since they were to be directed against magical causal agents. If he belonged to an Indian tribe in ancient central California, he would cut into a vein in the patient's right arm to wash away the demons that brought diseases of the arms and legs;

to be rid of those responsible for diseases of the torso, he cut into the veins in the left arm. Were he an Inca in long-ago Peru, he would cut a slit between the patient's eyes to release the demons of headache and madness. Were he a Koniaga Indian of Alaska or a Polynesian, he would have his people squeeze, rub, pummel, or wrestle a patient about day after day; in Hawaii, he would order weighty objects rolled over the patient; working anywhere in the world, he would likely sing chants and beat a drum or have his people raise a ruckus outside the patient's dwelling. Behind all these strategems was the hope of making life so uncomfortable for the demons that they would depart.

Were he a shaman, he would take another tack. He would put his mouth to the patient's body, suck out the causal agent, and then spit out a small stone, an insect, or a piece of wood or bone that he claimed had been somehow shot into the patient by an enemy. He did not brand himself a charlatan because he had secreted the object in his mouth beforehand. Nor did any patient who was aware of the subterfuge. By some unexplainable suspension of belief, both were convinced that the treatment was not a trick but a valid treatment that ended in a cure. Further (and it seems almost certain that autosuggestion was at work here), the patient would claim to have felt a sharp pain at the height of the procedure and then instant relief.

Using yet another magical tactic, the medicine man might elect to coax the demons out into the open with prayers, compliments, tasty foods, or special pleas, and then employ some ruse to be rid of them forever. Sir James Frazer, in *The Golden Bough*, provides a fascinating example of how this trickery has been put to work in the South Pacific. He writes that:

On the Indonesian island of Nias, when all efforts to drive off the demon of a given disease have failed, the medicine man pounds a small pole into the ground in front of the patient's house and extends a rope of palm leaves upward from it to the rooftop, after which he climbs to the roof with a pig and then rolls the animal off the roof. The demon now abandons the house via an opening in the roof and works his way down the rope to collect the succulent prize. Immediately, the medicine man calls upon a good spirit to prevent the demon from returning up the rope to the house and the patient. Should the strategy fail, the medicine man knows that more than one demon is at work. And so he sends a number of village men into the house and imprisons them by closing and locking all the doors and windows, leaving only the opening in the roof. Once securely locked in, the men begin to chant and beat drums and gongs in an effort to send the rest of the demons fleeing through the rooftop opening.

In another South Pacific ploy, the medicine man places bits of food on the patient's forehead and on a little doll lying close by, all in the certainty that the demon will emerge to nibble the food on the forehead and then, when done, will glimpse the tidbits on the doll and jump over to have a go at them. Still another strategy calls for the demon to be lured out of the patient and then sent to a distant place in a boat. It can be used to cure an individual or can be brought to bear on behalf of a village or an entire tribe when struck by an epidemic. For an example of how this works, we return to Indonesian waters:

> When suffering an epidemic, the people of the island of Ceram build a small ship, equip it with a sail, and load it with a cargo of rice, eggs, tobacco, and other enticing commodities. A specially chosen villager then shouts the news of the wonderfully provisioned vessel and begs the demon to go aboard and sail away with its riches. The ceremony ends with the ship and its passenger being put to sea, hopefully to travel far away and never to return.

The strategy is not unique to Ceram. Variations of it were practiced by a number of cultures in antiquity. For instance, the physicians of ancient Mesopotamia, who figure in the early history of formal medicine, often coaxed or tricked demons into a toy boat, which they would then set adrift on the Tigris or Euphrates. A similar tactic saw them pray the demons into a jar of water; the jar was then smashed on the ground so that the unwelcome visitors would flow away in the water.

Now let us turn to what the medicine man had to do when faced with a sickness caused not by invading demons but by the loss of that most vital of human possessions—the soul. To begin with, he knew that the soul could vanish in a number of ways. An angry god could take it. A spirit, a ghost, a demon, or a sorcerer (in this case, an evil magician and not the medicine man mentioned earlier or the Sorcerer of Les Trois Freres) could steal it. The device of an enemy (that rope dangling from a tree, for one) could snatch it away. And the soul was perfectly capable of wandering off by itself, with a number of peoples believing that it escaped for a night on the town via the nose or mouth while a person slept. Some were careful never to let infants sleep on their backs with their mouths open; some were quick to shut a sleeper's mouth whenever they saw it hanging open; some refused to disturb or move the sleeper if they thought his soul was away, for then the wanderer would never find its way back to its owner.

The medicine man also knew that his people believed, as many people still do today in primitive societies, that unless he acted quickly and successfully, the loss of the soul meant a swift death for the patient. Only in a few societies—among them the North American Flathead Indians—was there the view that the soul could wander off without death soon coming. But even then the soul had to be found and returned. Otherwise, death would certainly be the patient's eventual lot.

When dealing with a departed soul, the medicine man's treatment depended on where he was practicing. In the Celebes Islands of the Pacific, where the people believe that the soul has run away, he would order the patient to be beaten so that the soul would be shamed into returning. Were he a Dyak of Borneo, his fingers would be fitted with fish hooks for catching the soul as it flew away. Working among the Haida Indians of Canada and the northwestern United States, he would routinely carry a hollow bone in which the departing soul, on being captured, would be imprisoned until it was returned to its owner. Were he a shaman, he would first prowl the surrounding countryside for the departed soul;

should the search prove fruitless, he would enter a trance and descend to the underworld to meet the spirit enemies that had stolen or eaten the soul. He would argue—and often do battle—for its return.

The magical approach to treatment is both psychological and religious, and there is little doubt that medicine men through the centuries have understood this. But, of course, sickness is a physical problem, and so the medicine man has long wrought his magic in tandem with medications of supposed or genuine efficacy. The combination of the two approaches is easily seen in a number of African societies, where, as folklorist Bruce Jackson points out in *American Folk Medicine: A Symposium*, disease is seen as a religious experience. There, the medicine man, on assessing the cause and nature of a sickness, approaches the patient with a combination of physical and spiritual—or psychological—treatments. On the one hand, he employs such physical cares as massages and medications made of herbs, seeds, roots, juices, and minerals, while on the other, he brings to bear such psychological ammunition as prayers, magical leaps over the patient, and the call for his charge to avoid certain acts and foods or to sacrifice an animal, such as a goat or chicken. The combination is intended to help the patient physically and to convince him that all is going to be well from now on.

Physical treatments, from plant medications to surgeries, have played as important a role in the medicine man's practice as has magic with its attendant psychological values. From the preceding chapters, we know that the North American Indian medicine man employed a wide variety of plant cures: the buckeye for rheumatism and hemorrhoids, the mayapple as a laxative and a vehicle for aborting pregnancies, and the top leaves of the sage plant for coughs, colds, and tuberculosis. When magic played a part in the use of these plants, it usually did so in two ways. First, many of the plants were thought to have curative powers because they had been unearthed by magical beings, such as the spirits Bear and Badger, with their superb digging skills. Second, some medicine men, as did many doctors in the history of formal medicine, mixed into the plant medications disgusting ingredients meant to drive the demons of illness into flight by assaulting their sensitivities—ingredients that, as mentioned in earlier chapters, could include animal parts, human fingernail parings and hair, and human or animal feces.

In addition to the plant cures, the medicine man has also been long acquainted with procedures that have no magic attached to them whatsoever, even though the health problems requiring their use have been thought to have been caused by something magical, an evil spirit or an unknown enemy. In various societies, he long ago learned to cauterize wounds with hot ashes, heated blades, or chunks of iron. He learned to set broken bones in splints and casts of clay, and to coat infections and wounds with soothing mud and plant poultices. In prehistory, as you'll recall from chapter three, he successfully trephined the skulls of living patients to release the demons of headache or madness. The Ashanti medicine man in West Africa has long treated snakebite by first puncturing the affected vein with a knife, a splinter of bone or rock, or his version of a hypodermic needle—a small arrow shot into the vein—and then sucking out the venom through a bone tube or similar instrument. A remarkable method for suturing wounds is used by some Indian tribes in Brazil and was commonly practiced in ancient India and Africa: the suturing is accomplished by placing certain ants—the Bengali ant has long been a popular choice—on the wound; the ants, equipped with broad heads and caliper-like jaws, bite into the flesh to either side, at which time their bodies are snapped off, leaving the heads behind as surgical stitches.

Some medicine men have pretty much, if not completely, ignored magic. Among their number are the American Indian practitioners who have specialized in plant treatments and have become known as herb doctors. Most *curanderos* of the American Southwest, Mexico, and Central America have depended on extensive study and experimentation to master the intricacies of their profession and, in common with the modern doctor, are credited with being able to practice as a result of their education.

The Right to Practice

Since he practiced—and still practices—a medicine whose very name suggests the magical, the superstitious, and the primitive, the medicine man has too often been regarded with skepticism and a mild contempt by the modern era as a leftover from a scientifically ignorant past. These reactions are unmerited. While the medicine man has operated mainly in primitive societies, and while magic has always played a major role in his work, he has always been, at core, a fine professional, well-versed in both physical and psychological healing. And, almost without exception, he has been required to earn the right to practice. In some societies, his position has been hereditary, but in most, as in the case of the *curanderos*, he has undergone a long period of apprenticeship before ever hanging out his shingle. The experience of many an aspiring African medicine man is not unusual. He apprentices himself to a recognized practitioner for an extended period at an established fee, with the opportunity to move on to advanced—postgraduate—study if he wishes to and possesses the ability to delve deeper into the intricacies of his profession. The length of an apprenticeship, not just in Africa but anywhere, can run as long as fifteen to twenty years.

In addition to mastering the skills of his trade during his apprenticeship—everything from magical rituals and incantations to plant cures and surgeries—the apprentice must absorb a massive amount of knowledge about his people, their customs, their traditions, and their individual desires, fears, and needs. By the time he is ready to practice, he has become the counterpart of the family doctor in modern medicine—a physician able to treat a patient not simply on the basis of symptoms but also on an intimate understanding of the patient's personality, needs, and family history.

The apprenticeship makes other demands as well. While learning all possible about his people, the trainee must also coach himself to live apart from their everyday lives, for as long as he practices, he must remain aloof from his people, never letting them see his human weaknesses so that he will always keep their respect. Consequently, he is usually destined for a life without intimate friends. In some societies, he may not marry. In all, he must be the strongest, the wisest, and most mysterious, and the most spiritual man in view.

He must exhibit these characteristics because his people expect them of him. Throughout history, medicine men have always been individuals with a different tint to their natures. Some have shown an ability to go into trances and are thought to have been epileptics or to have been suffering from some other unknown malady. Some have been capable of an awesome energy while in a trance (a Tibetan community takes great pride in the medicine man who, on working himself into a spiritual frenzy, can run in a circle for nineteen hours nonstop). Some have survived a seemingly deadly accident or illness when young. Some have been homosexuals or transvestites. Some have been admired simply because they talked to themselves. And some have been burdened with some combination of these characteristics.

What is at stake here is a primitive mindset that is completely at odds with our own. We are inclined to pity the victims of horrendous illnesses and accidents and to shun characteristics and behaviors that are away from what we judge to be the norm. But not so a primitive people, who have eons of beliefs and customs embedded deep in their beings, all meant to help them survive in a mysterious world. They are awed by unusual personality traits and behaviors, and look on them as signs of their medicine man's contact with the realms of magic and the supernatural.

While the characteristics that set an individual apart from the general run of humanity make him a prime candidate for the post of medicine man, they do not alone qualify him for the post. As is customarily the case in formal medicine, some young people have become medicine men because it was their life's ambition. Others have been chosen for the work because they showed a natural skill in medical matters—the skill, for instance, to set broken bones or to mend torn flesh.

THE MEDICINE MAN AND HIS COMMUNITY

As holds true even today, the early medicine man was invariably far more than a physician. As one of the most distinguished members of the community, he was routinely called on to perform a variety of social, political, and religious functions. For one, he counseled parents on the rearing of their children and predicted what the future held for the young ones. For another, the magic that he employed for healing could also be marshaled to protect his community or any person within it from the evil intent of enemies (many primitives of the West Indies and the South Pacific remain convinced that their medicine man can put a "hex" on an enemy from miles away). For still another, he sat with the tribal chieftains and other officials when such matters as war and community problems were discussed; his opinions and advice were heard with respect. Not infrequently, he himself served as the tribal chieftain.

He also served as a religious leader, with some groups, such as the Omaha Indians of North America, looking on him as their direct contact with their gods. It was his job in many societies to lead his people in their various religious exercises—ceremonies that appealed to their gods to provide them with good harvests, successful hunts, and rain when it was needed.

Depending on where he lived, his harvest-time duties might require him to perform rites that would make it safe for the people to eat the crops they had grown. The need for these rites evolved from the belief that food on which the people depended for life came from a god or actually contained the god, and could not be consumed until a formal ritual won the deity's permission. Thus it is that a Brazilian tribe will not eat burgeoning maize until it has been ceremonially blessed; to do otherwise is to invite certain death. After carefully washing a half-ripe husk at harvest time, they place it before their medicine man, who then works himself into a frenzy by singing, dancing, and smoking for several hours. Finally, shouting in a fit of trembling ecstasy, he bites into the husk. The harvest of maize is now safe to eat.

Another of the medicine man's duties, which he performed periodically (often annually), called for him to conduct his tribe's purification rites. These rites, as their name indicates, are meant to cleanse the people of the contamination inherent in a wide range of substances. Chief among the contaminants most feared by primitives worldwide are blood, birth, and death. (You'll recall from chapter five the fear that many people, in both primitive and advanced societies, have felt since antiquity for the malevolent forces in menstrual, parturient, and placental blood. The same fear was often extended to blood spilled in an accident or in battle.) Depending on the people involved, a host of other items were long ago added to the list, including trees, rocks, certain foods and drinks, and even certain individuals.

Over the centuries, the methods of purification for individuals and tribes have proved to be almost as many as the contaminants themselves. They vary from tribe to tribe and from culture to culture. Some involve blowing smoke over the people. Some call for the people to jump over fires. Some demand that individuals or an entire community bathe. Some see all the homes in a village fumigated, all old utensils replaced with new ones, and all clothing burned. Some groups select a scapegoat that, taking on the burden of the community's contamination, is sacrificed or driven away. The scapegoat may be an object, an animal, or a fellow tribesman. The sacrifice may see the scapegoat thrown over a cliff, stoned to death, or exiled across a distant border.

FAITH HEALING

Without ever using the term itself, we have been talking about faith healing in this and other chapters. This is the belief that pain and disease can be neutralized through faith in a divine or supernatural power, and it has been with us since the dawn of time. It has been present in the work of every medicine man who has employed magical cures; his success has always depended on the patient's faith in him and his methods. It has been present down through the centuries in the trust that people over the world have placed in the curative and preventive powers of amulets, charms, and religious relics. It was present in the healing works of Christ and the Apostles and, later, in those of Martin Luther, the Quakers, the Baptists, and the Mormons. In our time, it has been present in the myriad healing miracles credited to the grotto at Lourdes and to St. Winifred's spring at Holywell in Wales. It remains with us today in a number of religions and philosophies, major examples being Unity, Theosophy, and Christian Science. Christian Science, however, maintains that healing comes not through faith alone but through the regeneration that comes with a true understanding of God.

There is, however, one aspect of faith healing that has yet to be mentioned—the inexplicable healing wrought by touch, by the simple "laying on of hands." Though practiced since antiquity and employed by some medicine men, this is not regarded as an integral part of the folk doctor's work (even the shaman, with the help he receives from the spirit world, does not cure by touch, but rather by the sucking process). Rather, most healing by touch has been the province not of medicine men but of blessed figures, individuals who have claimed to be blessed, and royal personages.

The most blessed of its practitioners was Jesus Christ, who performed several of his healing miracles by touch. Among the early royal figures said to have had healing powers in their hands were the emperors of ancient Rome. One of their number, Vespasian (A.D. 9–79) was reputedly able to heal with his foot. Legend holds that, with a single caress of his foot, he once healed a subject's crushed and torn hand.

Far better known than Vespasian as curers by touch were England's King Henry VIII (1491–1547) and his daughter, Elizabeth I (1533–1603). Both made their hands available to numerous petitioners of all classes, with Henry making a gift of 7s. 6d. to each person his hand graced.

But these two were latecomers to the art among western European royalty. Clovis of France (466–511) is said to have started the practice, with Edward the Confessor (1003–1066) following suit a half-century later in England. Edward, along with his reputation for curing all illnesses by touch, became especially famous for his ability to rid patients of scrofula (tuberculosis of the lymphatic glands, and, on occasion, the bones and joint surfaces). According to the twelfth-century historian William of Malmsbury, the monarch began touching for the illness when a woman told him of her dream that his hand could cure the disease in her. He responded by massaging her neck with his fingers after dipping them in water, with the woman then recovering quickly. The royal touch for scrofula spread throughout western Europe and remained in vogue until the eighteenth century. It was because of the belief that royalty could heal the condition that scrofula became popularly known as the King's Evil, or Queen's Evil if a woman happened to be occupying the throne.

Of the monarchs who cured the King's Evil, England's Charles II (1630–1685) ranks as the most ambitious. During his reign, he touched upwards of 100,000 patients. In 1684, he drew such a large and turbulent crowd for a "touching ceremony" that a half-dozen or so of the patients were trampled to death.

The practice started to go out of fashion soon after the death of Charles, when William III (1650–1702) bluntly damned it a "silly superstition." Queen Anne (1665–1714) was the last of Britain's "touching" mon-

archs. The nation's premier man of letters, Samuel
Johnson (1709–1784), once sought her help to be rid
of a case of scrofula. Her royal touch failed to be of
help.

The healing of the King's Evil and other illnesses by
touch has given the history of folk medicine some of
its most fascinating pages. The British long believed
that the royal possessions as well as the royal hand
could cure the Evil. One belief held that the water
from the well in which King James II (1633–1701)
cleansed his sword after the battle of the Boyne would
work. Another maintained that, if touched, a set of
underpants once owned by Charles I (1600–1649)
could do the trick. The King's Evil, plus a host of
other problems, among them sore throats, wens, and
warts, could be cured by pressing the hand of a corpse
against the troubled body part (especially the hand of
someone who had died an untimely death) or by touching a seventh son. Mention must also be made of the
many cures that were described in earlier chapters—
for example, healing a sty by rubbing it with gold or
dipping a wart into spunk water. All represent faith-
healing cures by touch.

Curing by the "laying on of hands" continues to
be practiced to this day. As was the case with their
predecessors, it is impossible to judge whether
modern-day touch-healers are actually blessed with
supernatural powers; whether their cures, if successful, are achieved through the powerful auto-
suggestion resident in all magical treatments; or
whether they are charlatans who prey upon the gullible and desperate with self-proclamations of completely absent skills. All that one can do is echo the

words that have been said about Lourdes and the many cures it has allegedly wrought: for those who do not believe, there is no explanation; for those who do believe, no explanation is necessary.

A GLOSSARY

More Cures and Curiosities

As its title suggests, this glossary is intended to provide points of extra interest. It contains entries of two different types. First, there are those on subjects that were omitted from the text to facilitate the flow of each chapter, a prime example being the medications, treatments, and objects that were used for so many different ailments that to have mentioned them with each malady would have led to a tiresome repetition. Second, there are entries that provide additional information on the topics mentioned in the chapters—peripheral information that, though interesting, ran the risk of digressing too far the subjects at hand and thus slowing the pace at which their stories could be told. Accompanying each such entry will be a reference to the chapter or chapters to which it pertains.

A

Amulets and Charms: Today, the terms *amulet* and *charm* are used interchangeably by most people (amulets are mentioned throughout the book, and charms in chapter four). Strictly speaking, however, there is a distinct difference between the two.

It is easier to explain the difference by beginning with the charm. With its name coming from the Latin word *carmen*, meaning "song," a charm is an incantation reputed to have magical powers. It is meant to bring a person, a family, a village, or a people good fortune and to protect against myriad dangers—among them illness, death, enemies, witches, and evil spirits. The incantation can take several forms. It can be a song, a prayer, a series of "mystical" words, or a chant. The charm can be said over potions and objects, such as necklaces, medallions, and even stones. The magic is passed to the potions and objects, and they themselves then become charms.

An amulet is an object that also protects one from the above dangers and serves to bring good fortune in all aspects of the owner's life. Usually small and often made of a durable substance, the amulet is customarily worn or carried on the body, secreted in one's possessions, or placed somewhere in the home. In many societies, it is common practice to equip barns, livestock, and fields with amulets to insure their well-being.

Over the centuries, amulets have been fashioned of an endless number of substances—metals, stones, minerals, animals and insects, plants and trees, animal and human parts (hair, claws, fingernails) and even animal and human urine and feces.

Three reasons account for amulets and charms being confusing and easily interchangeable terms. First, both promise the same wonders. Second, the word "amulet" is derived from the Latin *amuletum*, meaning "a charm." Finally, of course, the magical blessing that is a charm is often said over a potion or an object, with the magic power of the one being passed to the other.

B

Bezoar Stones: Bezoar stones are inorganic masses, often of magnesium phosphate and lime, that form around foreign substances in the alimentary organs of ruminants. They were once thought by a number of Old and New World societies to be both a gem and a medical marvel. They were mentioned in the writings of the ancient Persians and Arabians, were known to Europeans from the twelfth century onward, and were admired by the Chinese on one side of the Pacific and the American Indians on the other.

The stones served various purposes. The Sioux Indians blew bezoar dust into the eyes to strengthen both the sight and the intellect. In central Europe, the stones were swallowed to cure toothache. In Persia and India, they were employed as a laxative. Their greatest use, however, was as an antidote for poison. When taken internally, placed on a wound, or worn as an amulet, popular belief held that they were able to neutralize poisons. They found great favor among those figures—kings, politicians, and the wealthy—who most feared death by poisoning at the hands of ambitious and avaricious enemies. In time, with such a rich clientele at hand, the bezoars joined the most expensive medical safeguards on the market. In the 1700s, a stone could bring fifty times the price of an emerald.

Regardless of their reputation, the stones were distrusted by some of the best minds in medical history. The noted French surgeon Ambroise Paré (1510–1590), had no use for them, insisting that there was no such thing as a universal antidote for poison. To prove his point, he talked Charles IX into engaging in an experiment to prove their worthlessness. The king, whose trust in his own bezoar matched Paré's scorn for it, selected a criminal due to be hanged and had him given poison, after which the man was made to swallow a bezoar. The poor fellow spent seven hours dying—all the while retching, sweating, thirsting, and bleeding from the mouth, nose, and ears. Paré attempted to save the unfortunate's life, but failed. He wrote that the man "died miserably, crying it would have been better to have died on the gibbet." The experiment, however, so altered Charles's view of his own cherished bezoar that he had it burned.

The bezoars constituted just one type of several stones once reputed to contain mystical and medical properties. (See LEE STONE, LODESTONES, MOONSTONES, SNAKE STONES, and TOADSTONES.)

C

Catnip and a Rumor: For as long as it has been famous as a curative, catnip (see chapter one) has been notorious for the way it attracts and unhinges that aloof creature for which it is named. The source of the ecstasy here is the aromatic oil that the plant exudes to ward off insects. Cats quickly learn that the oil is released in increasing amounts when they rub against the plant and then—getting happier and dippier by the minute—roll about on it after knocking it down. All this feline hysteria started the word going round some years ago that catnip works as a mild hallucinogen in humans when smoked or taken in liquid. You can forget all the talk. Catnip unhinges cats, not humans.

D

The Doctrine of Signatures: This is a medical system grounded in the belief that all plants are created to serve humanity and that their specific curative values can be clearly seen in their God-given physical characteristics. For example, because of its bright yellow flowers and the orange color of its juice, the celandine plant was brought to bear against jaundice and other liver problems for centuries in Europe and elsewhere. Those same centuries saw the bladder-shaped pod of the Chinese lantern plant serve as a medication for facilitating urination and expelling kidney and bladder stones. The blossoms of the eyebright plant, which frequently remind one of bloodshot eyes, were long used to treat sore eyes and conjunctivitis, a job they did well because of the their anti-inflammatory properties.

Exactly when and how the Doctrine of Signatures first took shape is unknown. It may, however, have gotten its start with the ancient Chinese. At least a century before the birth of Christ, they noted that the root of the ginseng plant resembled the human figure and began advising its use for sharpening the mind, increasing wisdom, and achieving longevity (though its root was similar to that of the mandrake—see chapter four—they did not think of the plant as an aphrodisiac; that idea was left to other cultures). The doctrine was highly popular in Europe during the Renaissance and for several centuries thereafter, much due to the writings of its greatest proponent of the time, the Swiss physician and alchemist Paracelsus (1493–1541; born Theophrastus Bombast von Hohenheim). But, at a far earlier date, the Greeks may have practiced the doctrine to some degree. They used eyebright blossoms to treat failing sight and other eye problems. Eyebright's botanical name, *Euphrasia*, is derived from the Greek word meaning "good cheer." The name is thought to have been inspired by the happiness patients expressed when the plant improved their vision.

E

The Eucalyptus Tree as a Malaria Fighter: The medicinally valuable eucalyptus trees and bushes (see chapter one) come in more than five hundred varieties. One of the best-known of the lot is the blue gum tree. Along with its other curative tasks, it has long served as a malaria fighter. It does so not as a medicine but as a sponge. Its roots have a remarkable talent for absorbing water from the surrounding ground, and the tree has been planted in marshy areas in several areas of the world and has cleared them of the disease by depriving the malaria-carrying mosquitoes of a place to breed. Because of this talent, the blue gum is known as the Australian fevertree.

F

The Fig: In common with other foods, this native of western Asia and the Mediterranean regions was considered sacred by a number of ancient societies. In Rome, it was held sacred to Bacchus, the god of wine, and its milk was sacrificed to the goddess of fertility and birth, Juno Caprotina. The Timbuka people of Africa have long sheltered the spirits of their ancestors in the shade of revered fig trees. Buddhists regard one variety of fig tree (*Ficus religiosa*) as sacred because their Gautama Buddha is said to have been blessed with his divine powers while sitting beneath its leaves. The story of Jesus wishing to eat figs on his journey to Bethany caused the English of yesteryear to give the name Fig Sunday to Palm Sunday.

The fig's use as a medicinal and a health-giving food can be traced deep into antiquity. The Greeks fed its milk to infants and so valued the fruit itself as a staple that, at one point in their history, they abandoned it as a highly profitable trade commodity and outlawed its export. As did their ancestors, the Hindus in modern India and the people of several German and Austrian regions turn to the fig to ease toothache: in one German area, a dried fig held in the mouth is the traditional cure for a misbehaving tooth; elsewhere, the fruit is cooked in milk before being applied to the pained area. The Hindus also depend on the bark of the fig tree to cure diabetes. Other folk remedies call for the fruit to be mixed with grease and placed on the bites of mad dogs, and to be blended into concoctions meant to handle ailments that range from coughs and lung congestions to running sores and scrofula.

The Fish as Brain Food: Along with being considered an effective aphrodisiac (see chapter four), the fish has long enjoyed the reputation of being a brain food. This idea may have taken shape due to the animal's phosphorus content or its ability to swim through—penetrate—water, a facility that our forebears could easily have extended from an indication of sexual prowess to one of intellectual capacity. I've come across at least two stories of how this notion may have come into being. The first, as reported by Dr. Bruno Gebhard in *American Folk Medicine: A Symposium*, has it that the idea was born in the nineteenth century when German physiologist Jacob Moleschott (1822–1893) and a philosopher colleague—thought to be Ludwig Buchner (1834–1899)—passed on their admiration of phosphorus to the European public in the slogan "Without phosphorus—no thought." Gebhard goes on to mention a rhyme learned by American schoolchildren early in our century:

Fish is a brain food that is never said to fail,
I therefore recommend that you should eat a whale.

Dr. Gebhard then wryly notes that the rhyme gave birth to a widely-held misconception. The whale is not a fish.

The second story does not mention phosphorus and so may have more to do with the notion of "penetration." In *Man, Myth, and Magic*, Eric Maple writes that the fish most likely won its reputation as a brain food because the people of another day knew that it was a dietary mainstay for monks, who may have been disliked for their religious stands but were widely admired for their intellectual prowess. The truth of the matter, Maple points out, is not that the monks downed more than their fair share of fish but that they came mainly from the upper classes and thus had the advantage of better educations.

G

Garlic: Known affectionately as the "stinking rose" or contemptuously as stinkweed, garlic (see chapters six and seven) has long served the entire world as a medicinal plant, perhaps even since prehistoric times. The written record of its use dates back at least four thousand years in China, where it was employed against respiratory ailments and hypertension. In the centuries before the birth of Christ, the Sumerians were listing it among their medicinal drugs, and the Egyptians were using it to treat such disparate problems as tumors, headaches, and malfunctioning hearts. The fact that Greece's Aristotle (384–322 B.C.) was a philosopher and not a physician did not stop him from describing garlic as a fine spring tonic and a cure for hydrophobia. Rome's Pliny the Elder contended that it would cure more than sixty ailments. The American Indians brought it to bear against intestinal worms and snakebite. In times of plague in Europe, the people were advised to avoid falling ill by wearing necklaces of garlic; it has been suggested by a number of historians and folklorists, perhaps waggishly, that the tactic probably worked simply because the smell of the necklace kept people away from the wearers. As recently as World War I, military doctors used garlic juice to treat infected wounds.

Though some scientists argue that garlic does not perform all the medical wonders attributed to it, there is evidence that it contains antiseptic, antispasmodic, and antibacterial properties that make it effective in the treatment of a wide assortment of ailments, among them some types of influenza, strep and staph infections, typhus, enteritis, and dysentery.

While the medical history of garlic is interesting, the history of its other uses over time is downright fascinating. Roman soldiers, believing it to be the plant of their god of war, Mars, ate garlic for courage and strength before going into battle. Pliny wrote of the belief that a magnet lost its power when rubbed with or when placed in the same room with garlic. In Europe, there was once the belief that if an athlete munched on a garlic bulb during a footrace, not one of his competitors would be able to catch him. Throughout Europe and elsewhere, the plant was—and, in some regions, still is—credited with the ability to ward off any evil creature one cares to mention—demons, witches, unfriendly ghosts and spirits, and vampires. One could keep each at bay by wearing garlic bulbs in the clothing, hanging them from the neck, or tacking them up somewhere in the home. In the United States of yesteryear, an unwelcome suitor could likewise be kept at arm's length. The object of his affections had only to decorate a chunk of garlic with two crossed pins, bury it in the middle of a crossroads, and lure the unsuspecting young man into walking across the "grave." All his ardor would instantly vanish.

Gems: Because of their recognized monetary value and because of the mystical significance seen in their colors, precious and semiprecious stones were put to medical use from antiquity onward, with all serving the same purposes: they were brought to bear against poisons, leprosy, insanity, inflammatory diseases, bladder infections, and snakebites. Some were also used to protect against such region-wide ills as the plague and such everyday trials as nightmares and insomnia. In addition, certain gems served individual purposes and were the subjects of some unusual beliefs. For example:

Parents in ancient Greece gave their children the *carbuncle* to wear when swimming. It reputedly protected the youngsters from drowning.

In the Europe of the Middle Ages, many people thought the *diamond* able to render the wearer invisible. Also widely accepted in Europe and elsewhere for several centuries was the belief that a diamond, when worn somewhere on the body, would protect against poison and the plague. It was said to be capable of curing leprosy, insanity, and bladder problems. In one of its more mundane uses, it allegedly put an end to nightmares.

Hindus thought the *emerald* an effective laxative. All one had to do to relieve constipation was to look at the gem. Engravers in a number of countries kept an emerald close at hand during work hours, glancing at it now and again to ease eyestrain.

Medieval Europeans believed that *jade* safeguarded one against colic and kidney problems when applied to the side. This reputation gave the gem its name, which comes from the Spanish *piedra de ijada*, meaning "stone of the side." Jade is also known as nephrite, which is derived from the Greek *nephros*, "kidney." In the Orient, a mixture of powdered jade, dew, and rice is said to purify the blood and strengthen the muscles and bones. The North American Indians have long worn jade as an amulet to protect against snakebite and to cure various disorders, epilepsy among them.

Like the diamond, the *opal* had the reputation for rendering its wearer invisible; as a result, it became the patron gem of thieves. Though also credited with curing eye problems, it was widely associated with bad luck and death, especially in nineteenth-century

Spain. There, King Alphonso XII gave an opal ring to his bride on their wedding day, only to have her die a short while later. He passed the ring to his sister, who then died within a few days. Next, the ring went to his sister-in-law; she was dead before three months had passed. Astonished at the deaths, Alphonso decided to defy the fates and wear the ring himself. It was a fatal mistake. He died soon after putting the ring on his finger.

For centuries, the *ruby* ranked as a popular choice for staunching hemorrhages because of its blood-red color. It was also credited with the ability to end grief and suppress the evil effects of luxury.

In Rome during the 1400s, physicians prescribed *topaz* to ease and heal hemorrhoids. Centuries earlier, Saint Epiphanius (c. 315–402) credited topaz with emitting a milky-white fluid that cured rabies.

The Tibetans look on *turquoise* as a good-luck gem and believe that it guards against contagious diseases. In parts of India, bathers wear it on entering the water, saying that it safeguards them against snakes and boils. In Europe and elsewhere, from the thirteenth century onward, horsemen wore turquoise to protect themselves from falls.

L

The Lee Stone: This was another of the several stones said to contain magical healing powers (see BEZOAR STONES, LODESTONES, MOONSTONES, SNAKE STONES, and TOADSTONES). It differed, however, from all the others. While they were to be found in various countries, there was only one Lee stone in the world. It was also known as the Lee penny and was mentioned by Sir Walter Scott in his novel, *The Talisman*, when he wrote of Sir Simon Lockhart of Lee and Cartland. It seems that Sir Simon, while fighting the Saracens in the Holy Land, was given a coin with a small stone embedded in it. He was told that when the object was dipped into water, it would imbue the water with the power to stop bleeding and to effect a variety of cures.

The story may be no more than legend. But, according to Scott, the stone actually existed in the nineteenth century and was principally used to heal the bites of mad dogs. Thomas R. Forbes, in *American Folk Medicine: A Symposium*, writes that Scott seemed to have been skeptical of the thing's reputed efficacy. He quotes Scott as saying that since "the illness in such cases frequently arises from the imagination, there can be no reason for doubting that the water which has been poured on the Lee penny furnishes a congenial cure."

Forbes adds that the stone was once owned by the Lockhart family and that it was described as small, triangular in shape, and dark red in color. It was set in a coin known as a groat, with the family allowing both rich and poor access to it in times of need. On one occasion in the 1600s, it was loaned to the city of Newcastle under a bond of 60,000 pounds in the hopes of ending an epidemic of the plague there.

Leeching: When the Inca medicine doctor in ancient Peru cut a slit between the eyes of a patient to free the demons of headache (see chapter eight), he was employing an early version of bloodletting. The practice, which prevailed for centuries, was eventually nicknamed *leeching* because that ugly little animal, the leech, became a widespread vehicle for sucking the blood away. In time, the idea that bloodletting released the demons of disease was replaced by the theory that fever was a heating of the blood and could be eased by reducing the amount of blood in the body.

Leeches were not only placed on the patient's body to suck out his or her blood, but were also applied to bruised eyes. They did their work in Europe and the United States (where they were once applied to a feverish George Washington) until the late nineteenth century. They continue to be employed in the Orient, South America, Mexico, and a smattering of United States backwoods areas.

Bloodletting with the leech is thought to have burdened the physician of yesteryear with the insulting nickname that is still heard on occasion today: *leech*. Actually, the reverse is true. The leech is the one who received its name from the doctor. The term comes from the Old English *laece*, meaning "a healer" or "one who relieves pain." It was early applied to British physicians, and the practice of medicine itself was known for years as *leechcraft*.

Lodestones: Like BEZOAR STONES, MOONSTONES, SNAKE STONES, TOADSTONES, and the LEE STONE, these chunks of magnetite (oxide or iron) were credited with extensive healing talents. When worn with a ring or an amulet with a gold setting, a lodestone was thought able to strengthen the heart; when set in silver, it enhanced the eyesight and other senses. It was carried about in the pocket or worn as a ring or necklace to cure rheumatism and the gout; one gout cure called for the stone to be bandaged to the bottom of the foot, from whence it reputedly soaked up the pain.

In one of the stone's oddest uses, a suspicious husband turned to it to test his wife's faithfulness, either by placing it under her pillow or touching her head with it. If she immediately and passionately threw her arms about his neck, the husband knew she was chaste and faithful. But she was in deep trouble if the test ended with her being tossed out of their bed. No one knows why or how the test came into into being.

M

The Mole: If ever there was a paradoxical creature in folk medicine, it is this lowly animal. Its history from antiquity onward has been one of being thoroughly detested for its living habits and, at the same time, highly prized as a versatile curative. Many ancient societies abhorred the mole because it lives underground, in what was thought to be the realm of the dead. But the Greeks, the Romans, and the Persians greatly admired its ability to survive within the damp and choking earth, and to do so despite being assumed to be blind. Out of this admiration, thanks to the human mind's ability to make highly imaginative (though often mistaken) associations, came the belief that the animal held divine strengths and that they could be passed into the sick to bring a return of health. In time, the animal's repute as a curative spread to all of Europe, and from there to the New World. The mole's use in folk medicine persisted well into this century and continues to be practiced by some rural people.

Perhaps reflecting the loathing that the animal triggered in most people, many of the mole cures were out-and-out sickening. They required that the animal be sacrificed, with its blood or flesh then to be fed to or rubbed into the patient. Patients throughout Europe drank the mole's blood to cure epilepsy and drunkenness. Eastern Europeans smeared it on the body to heal scrofula. The French and the English massaged it into the skin to be rid of wens, warts, and felons. The French poured it into the ears of the deaf. As for its viscera, the Lithuanians, in an especially cruel practice, tore the animal in half and applied the still-warm parts to areas of the body suffering rheumatic pains.

The mole's blood also served in amulets, as did the paw. French mothers commonly made necklaces of string dipped in the blood and placed them around their children's necks to protect against epilepsy. It was also a common tactic in both Europe and America to avoid toothache and rheumatism by wearing a small sack containing the paw.

The Moon and Folk Medicine: One of the moon's chief links to folk medicine is seen in the ancient superstition that this heavenly body can cause insanity, a notion that may have substance, considering the increase that has been long noted in the rate of crime and violent acts at full moon. It was because of this old superstition that, on toying with the word "luna" long ago, we devised the term *lunatic*.

Another connection with folk medicine is seen in the many early cultures that associated the moon with death. For the Persians, and the American Indians, it was the home of their virtuous dead. Other cultures thought it to be the ship that carried the departed to their final resting place. In pre-Christian Europe, the Gnostics believed that it transported their dead to the sun.

Still other connections: many societies—among them Greece and Egypt—held that sleeping with one's face to the moonlight weakens the eyesight. An Eskimo woman in Greenland, where the moon is believed to be a male (in sharp contrast to most societies, which look on it as female because of its paleness and luminosity), will not sleep on her back without first taking the precaution of rubbing her stomach with spittle. Her husband does not like her to look directly at the moon; perhaps he, too, fears its maleness, but he insists that it will drive her mad. A longtime European and American superstition advises that a new moon should not be to your front when first seen. Otherwise, you're bound for a fall—perhaps physical, perhaps from grace. Many people believe that the moon, with its gravitational pull, influences the frequency and intensity of illness; ranked among them long ago was William Shakespeare, who wrote in *A Midsummer Night's Dream*:

> Therefore the moon, the governor of the floods,
> Pale in her anger, washes all the air
> That rheumatic diseases do abound.

And, for anyone suffering the problem of thin or thinning hair (see chapter two), there is this familiar but far less poetic folk advice:

> Have your hair cut at the new moon and it will grow out much better.

The same counsel holds true for beards.

Moonstones: These are pieces of whitish feldspar in which people thought they could detect the image of the moon. Their application was supposedly able to cure epilepsy and nervous tension. They were also said to bring good fortune to their owners and to engender tender feelings in lovers.

P

Patent Medicines: This is the name given to the many liquids, powders, and salves that, purporting to cure anything from a lack of energy to bad backs, sore throats, and kidney and liver problems, were much in demand in the United States and elsewhere from the 1700s to the opening decades of the twentieth century. Produced by legitimate physicians, pharmaceutical companies, quacks, and out-and-out charlatans, they were so named because of the patents their inventors secured for them.

The patent medicine trade began in the early 1700s, when a swaggering British sea captain, one Thomas Dover, decided to come ashore and become a doctor. Not bothering to take any medical training, he opened an office for himself and was soon announcing, long and loud, that he had invented a marvelous medicine. He guaranteed that it could relieve almost any ailment and ease the user's tensions. He called the concoction "Dover's Sweating Powder." It became known to several generations of customers simply as "Dover's Powder."

The ex-seaman was right about one thing. His concoction did ease tensions and did give one a feeling of well-being—as, indeed, it should have. The stuff was liberally sprinkled with opium, which had been used as a narcotic and painkiller since antiquity. The powder became so popular that dozens of imitations flooded the European and American markets during the next two hundred years. Some, such as "Mrs. Winslow's Soothing Syrup," were advertised for general complaints. Others, among them "Dr. Cole's Catarrh Cure," were aimed at specific disorders.

The first imitations contained just opium. Later, many patent medicines were laced with morphine (an opium derivative), codeine (an alkaloid associated with opium but weaker than morphine), and laudanum (tincture of opium).

The introduction of morphine and the hypodermic syringe in the care of the wounded during the Civil War contributed mightily to the wealth of the patent-medicine trade. The drug and the syringe—the one with its great ability to kill pain because it was a purer form of opium, and the other making administration of the drug more efficient—were seen as blessings by army hospitals north and south of the Mason-Dixon Line. What was not fully recognized at the time, however, was the potency of morphine's addictive powers.

So many veterans were left heavily addicted at war's end that morphine addiction was quickly christened "the soldier's disease." They turned to the patent medicines to ease the withdrawal symptoms that came of being deprived of the drug. It has been estimated that, by the close of the nineteenth century, the veterans—joined by other patent-medicine fans, patients, and abusers—brought the total of narcotic addicts in the

United States to 400,000, or approximately one in every four hundred citizens.

The addicts came from every walk of life, but they shared one thing in common. The public viewed them with sympathy, not as criminals or weaklings, but as the victims of various illnesses who were trying to relieve their conditions as best they could. As for the addicts themselves, they behaved accordingly. They looked on themselves as respectable people, doing their best to raise their families, earn a living, and take part in community affairs. The public attitude towards the addict did not begin to change until the early twentieth century, when the dangers posed by the opiates became so widely recognized and feared that physicians and the government began to take action to discourage and ban their use.

It must not be thought that all patent medicines contained addictive drugs. Mingled into some—as remains the case with many modern medications—were percentages of alcohol, while others were made of herbs of acknowledged therapeutic value. Some contained harmless ingredients that, while doing no real good, did no harm.

The patent-medicine trade sowed the seeds of some of the most famous companies in manufacturing the nation's food. The histories of the General Foods and Kellogg companies can be traced, respectively, to C. W. Post and Dr. John J. Kellogg. For decades, Post fought the coffee habit with his "Postum," claiming that coffee was responsible for ills that ranged from traffic and factory accidents to divorce and juvenile delinquency. Kellogg, who routinely wore a white outfit with his pet cockatoo perched on his shoulder, invented the world's first precooked cereal and put it on sale as a patent medicine.

Pliny the Elder: Certainly one of the most prolific of the world's authors, Rome's Pliny the Elder (see chapters three through six) was born Gaius Plinius Secundus sometime around A.D. 23. In his early years, he saw military service in Germany, Spain, and Gaul, and was for a time a ranking officer with the Roman fleet.

His fame as a scholar and writer rests much—though by no means solely—on his *Natural History*, a series of thirty-seven books, which he titled *Historiae Naturalis 37*. Attempting to embrace all the known science of the day, Pliny covers not simply the medical matters mentioned in our earlier chapters, but animal life, astronomy, botany, mathematics, mineralogy, nature, and zoology. While *Natural History* remains a masterpiece of intellectual prowess and stamina, it suffers as a work of science because the author did not limit its content to established fact, but included superstitious notions and even accounts of mythical and imaginary animals.

The eruption of Vesuvius on August 24, A.D. 79 cost Pliny his life. While he was staying with a friend on the southern shore of the Bay of Naples, his host's home was threatened with falling rocks and ash. Pliny escaped the home, but, weakened by the sulphur pouring into the atmosphere, was unable to travel beyond the volcano's reach. According to his nephew, the author Pliny the Younger (A.D. 61–113), his body was found three days later, lying on its side as if in sleep and preserved in the ash that covered it.

R

The Rain and Folk Medicine: The coming of rain has always produced physical and emotional upsets in humans. Of the aches and pains that can accompany an arriving rain, we have these comments from two distinguished writers and the British doctor-naturalist-amateur poet who developed the world's first workable smallpox vaccine, Edward Jenner (1749–1823):

> A coming storm your shooting corns presage,
> And aches will throb, your hollow tooth will rage.
> Sauntering in coffee house is Dulman seen;
> He damns the climate and complains of spleen.
>
> *Rain*
> Jonathan Swift (1667–1745)

> As old sinners have all points
> O' the compass in their bones and joints.
>
> Samuel Butler (1612–1680)

> Old Betty's nerves are on the rack.
>
> *Signs of Rain*
> Jenner

Responsible for the discomforts noted by the trio—plus those experienced by countless other individuals through the ages—are the rising humidity and falling barometric pressure that herald a coming storm. These actions, causing an opening of the pores and requiring an adjustment of organs and joints to the altering pressure, can induce both nervousness and physical pain. Not everyone is bothered by the two actions, but they do trouble many a body. Especially hard-hit are body parts that are aging or suffering some disorder or that have been injured or subjected to surgery. As comedian Henny Youngman has observed, even today the National Weather Service is twelve hours behind arthritis.

Animals are likewise affected, both emotionally and physically, by the rising humidity and descending pressure. Certain animals, such as the donkey, rooster, and peacock, begin to squawk and bray and are thought to be expressing their discomfort by doing so. Pigs have been seen to toss their snouts in agitation. Cattle are known to huddle in groups—possibly to ease their nervousness, possibly to better protect themselves from the elements. And, as one old axiom has it:

Dogs eat grass before a rain.

Some folklorists think this saying is nonsense, but admit that it might be be valid when applied to aged, rheumatic dogs. In pain and feeling ill because of what is occurring in the air around them, they may be instinctively turning to grass as a means of purging their discomfort by vomiting.

S

Snake Stones: These are magical stones first thought to heal snakebite and later believed to counteract other poisons, cure ague and whooping cough, assist dentition, and bring good luck. The respect for the stones is thought to have begun in the earth's warm regions, where snakes are at their most plentiful, and in time to have made its way to gentler climates via the world's early trade routes.

There were several kinds of snake stones. One type was said to be extracted from the head of a cobra. Legend has it that another was made of coiled snakes that had become petrified. Pliny the Elder, in his *Natural History*, writes of the stone that takes shape when masses of snakes coil together and form "rings about their bodies with the viscous slime which exudes from their mouths;" he goes on to speak of the druid belief that the hissing snakes eject the stones as eggs and then describes one he has seen as being "about as large as an apple of moderate size."

The legend of how yet another type was created seems to be an obvious variation of Pliny's account. It holds that the stone took shape when serpents breathed on a hazel branch and produced a blue stone ring emblazoned with the figure of a yellow snake.

In general, snake stones were held against or bound to the bitten flesh until they absorbed the venom. Some were said to fall away from the wound when they were saturated with the venom or when it had been fully extracted.

Some stones were undoubtedly bony substances or calcium deposits taken from snakes and other animals. Others, which were innocently mistaken for the genuine article or were counterfeited for sale by charlatans, were crystalline rocks with colors—usually green or gray—similar to those of reptiles. Still others are known to have been no more than glass-like beads.

For other stones with magical and medicinal properties, see BEZOAR STONES, LEE STONE, LODESTONES, and TOADSTONES.

* * *

Sneezing: For a variety of reasons, sneezing was once thought to be a mortal danger. In Africa, India, and Persia, and among some North American Indian tribes, the sneeze was thought to be a sign that evil spirits were abroad. The ancient Hebrews feared the sneeze because they thought a man sneezed once and then died. There was also the widespread belief in Europe that the soul was housed in the breath and that the sneeze, causing the mouth to open and the breath to be sharply exhaled, opened the way for the soul to escape the body—and once the soul was gone, so was life.

Out of these varied beliefs came the worldwide custom of responding to another's sneeze with a "God bless you," *Gesundheit* (German for "health"), or some other appropriate spoken wish. In the English-speaking world, the most familiar of the responses is, of course, "God bless you." St. Gregory (540–604) is credited with giving the saying to the language.

There was yet another reason for these blessings. It stemmed from that often-mentioned ancient belief—that much illness was caused by demons who lurked everywhere and attacked their human prey from the air. Causing the mouth to fly open as it does, the sneeze gave them the opportunity to enter the body and begin to wreak their havoc there. A variation of this is seen in the old Hindu belief that evil spirits enter the body via the nose, with the intake of breath before the sneeze making that entry all the easier.

Despite the widespread fear of its dangers, the sneeze was not universally hated. The Greeks considered it an omen of good things to come; their attitude was based on the legend of Penelope's prayers for the speedy return of her husband, Odysseus (also known as Ulysses), from his wanderings. When her son, Telemachus, sneezed at the close of the prayers, she looked on it as a sign that they would soon be answered—and, as matters turned out, they were. The Germans thought that a sneeze during a conversation meant that the preceding remark was true. Sneezing was highly fashionable in Europe during the seventeenth century, when snuff, which was manufactured of crushed tobacco, was routinely sniffed up the male nose, with the resultant sneeze thought to clear the head.

The sneeze is the subject of a rhyme similar to—and perhaps inspired by—the ''Monday's child'' poem that was mentioned in chapter five:

Sneeze on Monday, sneeze for danger;
Sneeze on Tuesday, kiss a stranger;
Sneeze on Wednesday, sneeze for a letter;
Sneeze on Thursday, something better;
Sneeze on Friday, sneeze for sorrow;
Sneeze on Saturday, see your true love tomorrow;
Sneeze on Sunday, your safety seek,
Or the Devil will have you the rest of the week.

T

Toadstones: Toadstones were believed to come from inside the heads of toads and were reputed to have various powers—to counteract poison, to heal the bites of spiders, snakes, and other venomous creatures, and to ease what Sir Francis Bacon called the ''Trevailes of Women.'' The stones, which were shaped and colored like the toads from which they were supposedly extracted, were worn for several centuries in Europe as rings and amulets. They eventually went out of style when people began to suspect, as did naturalist Thomas Pennant, (1726–1798), that each was really nothing more than "the fossile Tooth of the Sea-Wolf or some other flat-toothed Fish."

Prior to this loss of repute, the recommended way to obtain a stone of your own was to kill a large toad, bury it in an anthill, and let the ants devour its flesh. (See also BEZOAR STONES, LEE STONE, LODESTONES, and SNAKE STONES.)

W

Water: Water, as essential to life as it is, has for ages been the source of medical folk customs that range from those involving entire cultures to those benefiting the single family or the individual.

The former usually entailed the use of water in ceremonies aimed at bringing rain to the growing crops on which a people depend for their health and their very survival. The ceremonies are still seen worldwide, some complex and others quite simple. Representative of the complex ones is the rain dance of the United States, Jacarilla Apaches: based on an ancient tribal legend, it requires the village people to dance under the direction of four elders who represent four water animals—the salamander, turtle, crawfish, and frog—while concentrating on the need for rain and keeping time with a song chanted by a villager representing the legendary character, Old Man Salamander. Representing the simplest are the following from three distinctly different societies:

Buddhist priests seek to bring rain by pouring water into holes in their temple floors. This action symbolizes the rain sinking into the earth.

The rainmaker on the South Pacific island of New Britain begins his ceremony by wrapping the leaves of a vine in a banana leaf. He then moistens the leaf with water and buries it in the ground, after which he imitates the sounds of falling rain with his mouth.

A tribal rainmaker in northern Australia begins by singing a magical song at the edge of a pool. He next scoops up some of the pool water, sloshes it about in his mouth, and spits it out, turning in various directions as he does so. He completes the ceremony by splashing water all over himself and scattering it about, after which he quietly returns to his home.

Water has been utilized for centuries by families and individuals as a folk curative for various ills. It was once the custom in the British Isles to cure thrush (a fungal infection that, characterized by whitish spots in the mouth, strikes infants and, occasionally, adults) with water from a southward-running stream. The cure could be achieved in any of several ways, with one popular method being to pull three rushes from a stream, pass them separately through the patient's mouth, and then toss them back in the stream, all in the faith that the thrush would sail away with them.

Whooping cough was also treated with a porridge

made over the water in a southward-running stream. Cold water from a stream or a well and placed in a bucket beneath a patient's bed was said able to heal bed sores and ease cramps. Holy water had a reputation for easing pain when massaged into the afflicted area.

Bibliography

Adamson, H.E., *Anthropology: The Study of Man* (3rd Edition). New York: McGraw-Hill, 1966.

Anderson, J. Q., "Magical Transference of Disease in Texas Folk Medicine," *Western Folklore*, July, 1968.

Armstrong, D. and E., *The Great American Medicine Show*. New York: Prentice Hall/Simon & Schuster, 1991.

Barkham Burroughs' Encyclopaedia of Astounding Facts and Useful Information 1889. New York: Bonanza Books, 1983.

Batchelor, J. F., and De Lys, C., *Superstitious? Here's Why*. New York: Harcourt, Brace, 1954.

Berry, P. D., and Repass, M. E., *Grandpa Says . . . Superstitions and Sayings*. Louisa, Kentucky: Printed by Billingsley Printing and Engraving, Fredericksburg, Virginia, 1980.

Blumenthal, S., *Black Cats and Other Superstitions*. Milwaukee: Raintree, 1977.

Bohle, B., *The Home Book of American Quotations*. New York: Dodd Mead, 1967.

Bombaugh, C. C., *Gleanings for the Curious from the Harvest Fields of Literature: A Melange of Excerpta*. Hartford, Connecticut; Cincinnati; and St. Louis: A. D. Worthington and A. G. Nettleton Companies, 1875.

Bremness, L., *The Complete Book of Herbs*. New York: Penguin, 1988.

Cavendish, R., editor, *Man, Myth & Magic: An Illustrated Encyclopedia of the Supernatural* (24 volumes). New York: Cavendish Corp., 1970.

Doane, N. L., *Indian Doctor*. Charlotte, North Carolina: distributed by Aerial Photography Services, 1980–1985.

Dolan, E. F., *Animal Folklore: From Black Cats to White Horses*. New York: Ballantine Books, 1992.

Dorland's Illustrated Medical Dictionary. Philadelphia and London: Saunders, 1988.

Dwyer, B., *2001 Southern Superstitions*. Highlands, North Carolina: The Merry Mountaineers, Inc., 1978.

Ehrenreich, B., and English, D., *Witches, Midwives, and Nurses: A*

History of Women Healers. New York: The Feminist Press at The City University of New York, 1973.

Emrich, D., *Folklore on the American Land*. Boston: Little, Brown, 1972.

Evans, I. H., editor, *Brewer's Dictionary of Phrase and Fable*. New York: Harper & Row, 1981.

Fergussen, R., *The Penguin Dictionary of Proverbs*. Hammondsworth, Middlesex, England: Penguin Books, 1983.

Fisher, M. F. K., *A Cordiall Water: A Garland of Odd & Old Receipts to Assuage the Ills of Man & Beast*. San Francisco: North Point Press, 1981.

Fletcher, S. E., *The American Indian*. New York: Grosset & Dunlap, 1954.

Frazer, J. G., *The Golden Bough: A Study in Magic and Religion* (Abridged Edition). New York: Macmillan, 1951.

Gaffney, S., and Cashman, S., editors, *Proverbs and Sayings of Ireland*. Portmarnock, County Dublin, Ireland: Wolfhound Press, 1974.

Gillette, F. L., and Ziemann, H., *The White House Cook Book*. Chicago: The Werner Company, 1887.

Graves, R., *The Greek Myths: Volume 1*. Baltimore: Penguin Books, 1955.

——*The Greek Myths: Volume 2*, Baltimore: Penguin Books, 1955.

Haggard, H. W., *Devils, Drugs, and Doctors: The Story of the Science of Healing from Medicine-Man to Doctor*. New York: Harper & Row, 1979.

Hand, W. D., editor, *American Folk Medicine: A Symposium*. Berkeley: University of California Press, 1970. The following is a list of the chapters researched, with the names of their authors:

    Brandon, E., "Folk Medicine in French Louisiana."

    Fife, A. E., "Birthmarks and Psychic Imprinting of Babies in Utah Folk Medicine."

    Forbes, T. R., "The Madstone."

    Gebhard, B., "The Interrelationship of Scientific and Folk Medicine in the United States of America since 1850."

    Hand, W. D., "The Mole in Folk Medicine: A survey from Indic Antiquity to Modern America II."

    Jackson, B., "The Other Kind of Doctor: Conjure and Magic in Black American Folk Medicine."

    Lacourciere, L., "A Survey of Folk Medicine in French Canada from Early Times to the Present."

    Myerhoff, B. G., "Shamanistic Equilibrium: Balance and Meditation in Known and Unknown Worlds."

    Talbot, C. H., "Folk Medicine and History."

    Vogel, J. V., "American Indian Foods Used as Medicine."

Harrowven, J., *The Origins of Rhymes, Songs, and Sayings*. London: Kaye and Ward, 1977.

The Illustrated Encyclopedia of Mankind. London: Marshall Cavendish, Ltd., 1978.

Jarvis, D. C., M. D., *Folk Medicine*. New York: Ballantine Books, 1982.

Jensen, Dr. B., *Foods that Heal*. Garden City Park: Avery Publishing Group, 1988.

Jobes, G., *Dictionary of Mythology Folklore and Symbols* (two volumes). New York: Scarecrow Press, 1962.

Johnson C., *What They Say in New England*. New York: Columbia University Press, 1963.

Kiev, A., *Curanderismo: Mexican-American Folk Psychiatry*. New York: Free Press, 1968.

Kowalchik, C., and Hylton, W. H., editors, *Rodale's Illustrated Encyclopedia of Herbs*. Emmaus, Pennsylvania: Rodale Press, 1987.

Kusinitz, M., *Folk Medicine*. New York: Chelsea House, 1992.

Leach, M., editor, *Funk & Wagnall's Standard Dictionary of Folklore, Mythology, and Legend*. New York: Funk & Wagnall's, 1984.

Lee, A., *Weather Wisdom*. Garden City: Doubleday, 1977.

Lund, D. R., *Early Native American Recipes and Remedies*. Staples, Minnesota: printed by Nordell Graphic Communications, 1989.

Magic and Medicine of Plants. Pleasantville, New York: The Reader's Digest Association, 1986.

Malinowski, B., *Magic, Science, and Religion, and Other Essays*. New York: Free Press, 1948.

Mindell, E., *Earl Mindell's Herb Bible*. New York: Simon & Schuster, 1992.

New Larousse Encyclopedia of Mythology. New York: Crescent Books, 1989.

Opie, I., and Tatem, M., *A Dictionary of Superstitions*. Oxford, England, and New York: Oxford University Press, 1989.

Panati, C., *Extraordinary Origins of Everyday Things*. New York: Harper & Row, 1987.

Perl, L., *Don't Sing Before Breakfast, Don't Sleep in the Moonlight: Everyday Superstitions and How They Began*. New York: Clarion Books, 1988.

Phillips, P. C., *Medicine in the Making of Montana*. Missoula: The Montana Medical Association and Montana State University Press, 1962.

Pickard, M. E., and Buley, R. C., *The Midwest Pioneer: His Ills, Cures & Doctors*. Crawfordsville, Indiana: R. E. Banta, 1945.

Pierce, R. V., M. D., *The People's Common Sense Medical Adviser in Plain English; or Medicine Simplified.* Buffalo: World's Dispensary Medical Association, 1895.

Radford, E., and M. A. (edited and revised by Christina Hole), *Encyclopedia of Superstitions.* London: Hutchinson of London, 1961.

Robinson, H. S., and Wilson K., *Myths and Legends of All Nations.* Garden City: Doubleday, 1960.

Schwartz, A., *Cross Your Fingers, Spit in Your Hat.* Philadelphia: J. B. Lippincott, 1974.

Smith, W. G., *The Oxford Dictionary of English Proverbs.* London: Oxford University Press, 1970.

Steele, P. W., *Ozark Tales and Superstitions.* Gretna, Louisiana: Pelican, 1988.

Stevenson, B., *The Home Book of Proverbs, Maxims and Familiar Quotations.* New York: Macmillan, 1948.

Tallman, M., *Dictionary of American Folklore.* New York: Philosophical Library, 1959.

Thomas, M., *Grannie's Remedies.* New York: Gramercy Publishing, 1965.

Vogel, V. J., *American Indian Medicine.* Norman: Oklahoma: University of Oklahoma Press, 1970.

White, M., "Alphabetical Folklore of Herbs," *The Old Farmer's Almanac,* 1992.

Wigginton, E., *The Foxfire Book.* Garden City: Anchor Press/Doubleday, 1968.

Wilen, L., and J., *Chicken Soup and Other Remedies.* New York: Fawcett, 1984.

Index

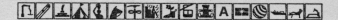

Also by

EDWARD DOLAN